# EXERCISE AND CORONARY HEART DISEASE

# EXERCISE AND CORONARY HEART DISEASE

## ROLE IN PREVENTION, DIAGNOSIS, TREATMENT

*By*

### GERALD F. FLETCHER, MD

*Director of Internal Medicine and Cardiac Rehabilitation*
*Georgia Baptist Hospital*
*Associate Professor of Medicine*
*Emory University*
*School of Medicine*

*and*

### JOHN D. CANTWELL, MD

*Director of the Preventive Cardiology Clinic*
*Atlanta, Georgia*
*Associate Director of Cardiac Rehabilitation*
*Georgia Baptist Hospital*
*Clinical Instructor in Medicine*
*Emory University*
*School of Medicine*

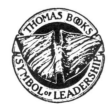

**CHARLES C THOMAS • PUBLISHER**
*Springfield • Illinois • U.S.A.*

*Published and Distributed Throughout the World by*
CHARLES C THOMAS • PUBLISHER
Bannerstone House
301-327 East Lawrence Avenue, Springfield, Illinois, U.S.A.

*With THOMAS BOOKS careful attention is given to all details of
manufacturing and design. It is the Publisher's desire to present books that
are satisfactory as to their physical qualities and artistic possibilities and
appropriate for their particular use. THOMAS BOOKS will be true to
those laws of quality that assure a good name and good will.*

**Library of Congress Cataloging in Publication Data**

Fletcher, Gerald F    1935-
  Exercise and coronary heart disease.

  1. Coronary heart disease.  2. Heart—Diseases—Prevention.  3. Exercise
—Physiological effect.
I. Cantwell, John D., joint author.  II. Title.
[DNLM: 1. Coronary  disease.  2. Exercise  test.  3. Exercise  therapy.
4. Exertion.  WG300  F612ea  1974]
RC685.C6F55      616.1′23′0624      73-21986
ISBN 0-398-03089-8

*Printed in the United States of America*

iv

To the Department of Medicine and the Cardiac Rehabilitation Staff at Georgia Baptist Hospital (both full-time and volunteer) for their success in developing and maintaining an effective inpatient and outpatient program for patients with recent myocardial infarction.

G.F.F.

To Marilyn, Brad, Kelly and Ryan—for love, happiness, and the joie de vivre.

J.D.C.

# CONTENTS

# PREFACE

CORONARY ATHEROSCLEROTIC HEART DISEASE (herein referred to as coronary heart disease) is pandemic in much of the world, especially in the United States where it claims the lives of over 700,000 persons annually; 40 to 50 percent of these persons never reach a hospital. This disease alone is the cause of 40 percent of all deaths. It is largely due to the frequent occurrence of coronary heart disease that American men rank eighteenth on a worldwide list of life expectancy. Coronary atherosclerotic disease frequently develops early in life as evidenced by autopsy studies of American men killed in the Korean War,[1] British pilots killed in air crashes,[2] and Chilean men and women who died in automobile accidents.[3]

Our current efforts to control this disease are divided into four general categories—prevention, diagnosis, treatment and rehabilitation. The purpose of this book is to consider the role of exercise and physical training in these four categories. For years exercise has either been overemphasized or underrated; it now becomes necessary to separate facts from fads as significant animal and human data begin to be reported.

In the area of coronary *prevention* we will identify the more significant coronary risk factors and consider the effect of exercise training on each factor. In terms of *diagnosis* of coronary disease, we will review the use of exercise stress testing and present data on various methods of testing that are applicable to patients who are either high coronary risks or who already show manifestations of the disease. We will consider the use of exercise as a *therapeutic* agent in coronary disease, both for inpatients and outpatients, and will outline and relate preliminary results of such specific programs. Lastly we will discuss the role of exercise in the *rehabilitation* of patients with recent myocardial infarction. In addition, we will also summarize the results of other investigators who have prescribed exercise for such patients and discuss the hemodynamic findings as well as the possible risks and complications involved.

It is our sincere hope that this book will be of particular use to the practicing physician, for it is he to whom the patient turns for medical advice regarding exercise, it is he who will need to advise the type and degree of exercise, and it is he who will share in the ultimate consequences.

ix

# ACKNOWLEDGMENTS

WE WOULD LIKE to express our appreciation to Barbara Johnston, M.N., and Fay E. Evat, Medical Librarian, for their contributions in research and acquisition of background material, to Mary Lewis, Neaka Kooken and Kay Watkins for editorial assistance and typing, to Martha Tarrant and Patsy Bryan for assistance in art work and illustrations, to Bob Beveridge for photography, to members of the Georgia Baptist Cardiac Rehabilitation team for their personal efforts in patient care and to the members of the outpatient gym exercise program for their enthusiasm and perseverance in properly-prescribed physical training.

G.F.F.
J.D.C.

# EXERCISE AND CORONARY HEART DISEASE

*Chapter I*

# HISTORICAL ASPECTS OF

# EXERCISE AND

# CORONARY HEART DISEASE

THE ARCHIVES OF ancient history have referred to the effects of exercise on many occasions. In 106 to 43 B.C., Cicero stated, "exercise and temperance can preserve something of our early strength even in old age." [4] Timaeus said of the body: "by moderate exercise reduces to order according to their affinities the particles and affections which are wandering about." [5] Richard Steele (1672 to 1729) stated, "reading is to the mind what exercise is to the body" [6] and Addison (1672 to 1719) said, "exercise ferments the humours, casts them into their proper channels, throws off redundancies, and helps nature in those secret distributions, without which the body cannot subsist in its vigour, nor the soul act with cheerfulness." [7]

Using exercise to improve the cardiovascular system and to promote longevity has been debated for many centuries. Chauncey Depew, who lived for ninety-four years, once stated, "I get my exercise acting as a pallbearer to my friends who exercised." [8] Easton, however, in 1799, reported 1,712 instances of longevity over one hundred years of age and remarked, "It is not the rich and the great, not those who depend on medicine, who become old: but such as use much exercise. For an idler never attains a remarkable great age." [9]

Exercise, as an adjunct to good physical health, attained popularity early in American history. In 1785, Thomas Jefferson, while minister to France, wrote to his nephew: "Walking is the best possible exercise. Habituate yourself to walk fast without fatigue." [10] In 1854, concerning treatment of fatty degeneration of the heart, Stokes said that a person must adapt to early hours and graduated exercise. [5]

During his influential years Doctor Paul Dudley White [11] has

3

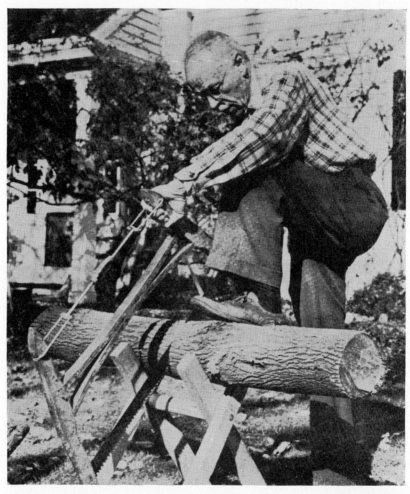

Figure  1.  Photo showing Dr. Paul Dudley White in his seventies perform-
         ing one of his favorite pastimes—"sawing logs" (Copied with
         courtesy from *Cardiovascular and Metabolic Diseases,* December
         3, 1973.)

referred to our easy way of living as a "real pity." He felt that our
ancestors were in better physical health because of their active
lives spent in clearing the forests and plowing the land. He felt
that exercise was the "best tranquilizer there is." In farewell comments to his many friends and acquaintances he was known to never

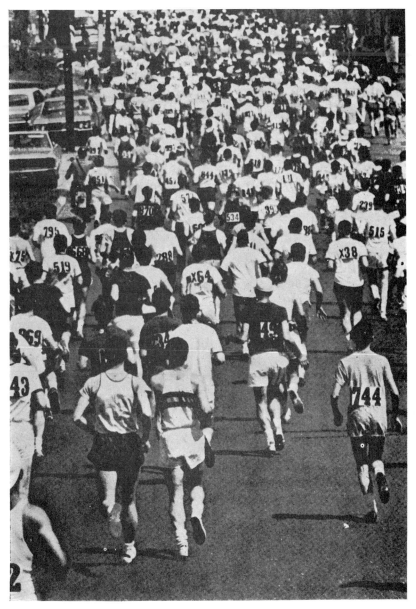

Figure 2. Photo showing group of runners in Boston Marathon, an event in which Clarence DeMar participated on numerous occasions.

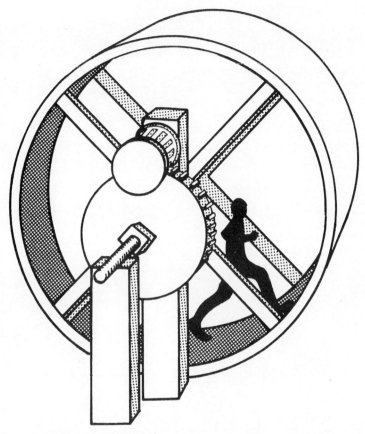

Figure   3.  Artist's sketch of a squirrel cage treadmill used for pumping
          (Borckler, G.A. Theatrum machinarium novum. Cologne, 1662.)
          Courtesy of the British Museum.

say "take it easy," but rather to say "take it hard." Dr. White is
shown in Figure 1 performing one of his many active exercise
habits.

Over the years it has become generally accepted that those persons who have physically active occupations enjoy better physical
health; such an assumption, however, is not totally supported by
sound evidence. Isolated case histories such as that of Clarence
DeMar,[12] the marathon runner of the early 1900's, provide striking
examples of the benefits of long-term physical conditioning. DeMar

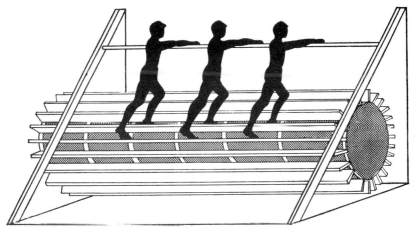

Figure 4. Artist's sketch of the treadmill at Brexton Prison.[13]

participated in marathon races (such as seen in Figure 2) for forty-nine years, and at his death (of metastatic rectal cancer) at age seventy, his coronary arteries at autopsy were two to three times the normal diameter.

One of the most important aspects of exercise activities has been that of "testing" the individual. Utilization of walk tests, step tests and treadmill tests are means by which normal and cardiac patients are evaluated for their safe exercise limits.

Historically, the Chinese, Romans and Greeks first used the treadmill for irrigation and construction projects over 2,000 years ago.[8] In 1818, William Cubitt, a British civil engineer designed an elongated "stepping wheel" on which dozens of prisoners could work side by side. In accord with this, treading-the-wheel for punishment became prevalent throughout English prisons. (Figures 3 and 4 show examples of "treading" used for punishment.) In 1846, however, because reformers considered treading-the-wheel a cruel, inhumane and unhealthy practice, Edward Smith began to investigate physical performance by utilizing new physiologic techniques during treadmill exercise.[13] These studies were the first systematic inquiry into the respiratory and metabolic response of the human to muscular exercise, and laid the groundwork for the extensive studies that have followed in the evaluation of exercise performance in patients with coronary heart disease.

Smith's early studies include measurements of inspired air, respiratory rate, respiratory stroke volume, pulse rate and oxygen production. By 1857, measurements were made for other types of exercise including swimming, rowing and horseback riding.[14]

With the acquisition of exercise habits early in history and the insight into methods of evaluation of exercise performance, observations [15] began to reveal in some instances a higher mortality rate in people with sedentary occupations compared to those who were physically active. These observations were to be the forerunners of more studies relating physical inactivity and mortality and morbidity from coronary heart disease.

As history has been influential in other fields of medicine, it appears that such trends have also developed in the relation of exercise to coronary heart disease. Although little or no specific mention is made of coronary heart disease in the aforementioned paragraphs, it can be assumed that, as is certainly true today, a considerable percent of human mortality was secondary to diseases of the heart and blood vessels—especially coronary disease. Sudden death has been a subject of recent interest; this most likely was prevalent in early history and, as is thought to be true today, was likely related in many instances to undiagnosed coronary atherosclerotic disease.

As the following chapters unfold to relate various aspects of exercise in the management of coronary heart disease, the reader should keep in mind the many historical aspects of exercise and good health. The scientific approach to prescribing the proper quantity and quality of exercise for the patient with coronary heart disease should be considered as a progressive extension of basic historical concepts.

*Chapter II*

# EXERCISE PHYSIOLOGY

# IN NORMALS AND IN

# PATIENTS WITH CORONARY

# HEART DISEASE

IN DEALING WITH patients, we, as physicians, are obligated to consider what goals we are trying to attain through exercise, and what parameters we are trying to achieve in the cardiovascular system.[16] These goals should be made clear when we discuss exercise with our patients, and they should be provided with a basic understanding as to how the normal and abnormal cardiovascular systems respond to exercise.

The external stress that may be imposed on the human body through some types of exercise may not actually alter the work of the heart itself or enhance "conditioning" of the cardiovascular system. For example, gardening, raking leaves, mowing grass and household domestic chores are types of exercise that individuals cannot refer to as "good exercise." These types of activity may impose fatigue and musculoskeletal strain on a subject, but do not necessarily cause high caloric expenditure. There is also a possible harmful isometric effect as will be later elaborated on in this chapter. To the contrary, jogging, swimming, brisk walking and sprinting cause higher levels of caloric expenditure and are considered dynamic and more efficient types of exercise. The calories expended per hour for various types of physical activity are listed in Figure 5 where data is taken in part from Falls.[17] Similar information is seen in Figure 6 which is the work classification scheme of Wells *et al.*[18]

## *Normals*

Regarding the cardiovascular system in recommending exercise and evaluating exercise, one should consider those factors that determine the work done by the heart, that is the *myocardial oxygen consumption*. Sarnoff *et al.*[19] and Monroe *et al.*[20] have clearly

9

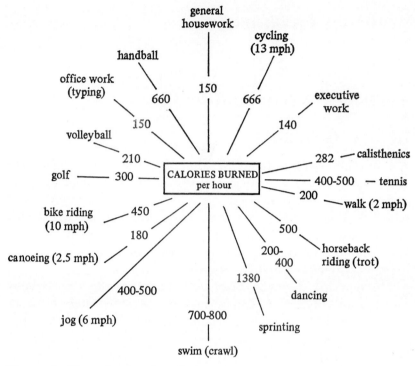

Figure 5. Chart showing the calories utilized per hour for various types of physical activity.

shown through precise physiological measures that heart work or myocardial oxygen consumption is directly related to the heart rate, systemic systolic blood pressure or intraventricular pressure and the inotropic or contractile state of the myocardium. These principles were transposed to the clinical setting quite vividly some years ago through the work of Robinson.[21] He found, in his group of fifteen patients with angina pectoris exposed to various types of progressive exercise training followed with periodic exercise testing, that the threshold at which pain developed was always related to a fixed level of systolic blood pressure and heart rate. Regardless of the increased duration of the exercise or the work load reached on the treadmill, the work level that precipitated angina pectoris in his patients was always at the same heart rate and systolic blood pressure.

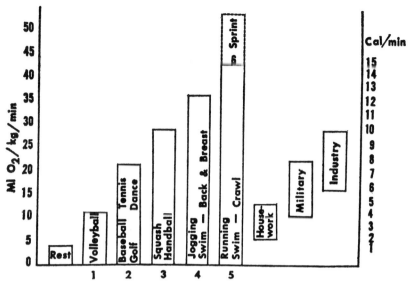

Figure 6. Bar graph showing oxygen consumption (milliliters per kilogram per minute) related to calories expended per minute for various levels of physical activity. The graph is from the work classification scheme of Wells *et al.*[18] (With permission of Harold B. Falls, Ph.D., from the *Journal of the South Carolina Medical Association, 65,* 1969, p. 8.)

The *circulatory dynamics* of exercise have been of interest for many years. In 1957, Mitchell *et al.*[22] related evidence that maximal oxygen intake is a measure of cardiac capacity and the ability to increase the arteriovenous oxygen difference, not of the ability of the vascular bed to accommodate left ventricular output. Because of this they felt that maximal oxygen consumption had clinical usefulness in evaluating patients with cardiovascular disease. In 1963, Frick *et al.*[23] studied fourteen young men with sedentary habits. After a two-month period of intensive physical training they found that eleven of the fourteen subjects had an increase in heart volume, higher cardiac output at rest and reduced heart rate at rest. During exercise and after a period of physical training, three subjects had a larger stroke volume and significantly lower heart rate. In 1968, Saltin *et al.*[24] studied five young normals extensively in a longitudinal study lasting three months. During the bed rest period of twenty days there was a pronounced decrease in maximal oxygen uptake, stroke volume and cardiac output. At the end of a following fifty-five day training period, two previously trained subjects were able to attain the same level of maximal oxygen uptake as they had reached in the initial control studies. Three previously sedentary subjects reached levels after training that were higher than their control values. In these latter three subjects the increase in maximal oxygen uptake after training was attributable to an increase in stroke volume and to widening of the arteriovenous oxygen difference. In addition to these aforementioned apparent hemodynamic benefits of training in normal young people, similar studies from the same laboratory by Siegel *et al.*[25] have shown a maximal oxygen uptake increase of 19 percent in nine healthy, blind sedentary men who participated in a fifteen-week quantitative physical training program.

Studies on older physically well-trained individuals have shown, in contrast to younger normals, that aerobic work capacity decreases with increasing age.[26] This is a basic principle to be aware of when testing individuals in the older age group, especially because of their statistical predilection to coronary disease.

### Heart Disease

Regarding studies in cardiovascular hemodynamics in patients with heart disease, a number of authors have related their experiences. Naughton *et al.*[27] in 1966, studied twenty-four men with well documented myocardial infarctions; twelve participated in a physical conditioning program and the remainder remained sedentary. After eight months the trained cardiac patients had significant training effects as reflected by the systolic and diastolic blood pressure and heart rate during rest, standing and comparable levels of energy expenditures. The response of the cardiac patient to that of a group of healthy normals indicated that the presence of disease did not necessarily affect the physiologic response of the subject.

In 1966, Varnauskas *et al.*[28] investigated the hemodynamic and metabolic effects of physical training in nine patients with coronary disease. In addition to clinical improvement after training they reported a hemodynamic adjustment toward a hypokinetic state and reduction in work of the left ventricle. Later in 1968, Frick *et al.*[29] assessed the hemodynamic effects of physical training in seven patients after myocardial infarction. The training was followed by a reduction in exercise heart rate and tension time index, enhanced stroke volume and improved left ventricular function. Concomitant with these hemodynamic changes exercise tolerance was improved.

More recently, Clausen *et al.*[30] studied the effect of physical training on the distribution of cardiac output in patients with coronary artery disease. This was done by measurement of cardiac output and regional blood flow parameters in liver and skeletal muscle at rest and during exercise. In seven of these patients, reported values were taken during a physical training program of four to ten weeks duration. After training, cardiac output was reduced at moderate work loads (13.1%) but increased (5.5%) during heavy exercise. Similar changes were seen in muscle blood flow which was decreased at submaximal loads (14.9%) and increased at maximal (8.6%). Hepatic blood flow showed, in contrast, a less pronounced reduction at both work loads after training (difference 7.2%). They felt that these noted effects of training could be explained as peripheral regulatory alterations without implying primary improvement in cardiac performance. They suggest that local changes in trained muscles are important for the reduction in myocardial pressure work caused by physical conditioning.

Detry *et al.*,[31] in 1971, reported the results of training in twelve patients with coronary heart disease. The rate-pressure product and the left ventricular work decreased after training, whereas stroke volume was unchanged and arterio-mixed venous oxygen ($A\text{-}V_{O_2}$) difference increased. The classic post-training bradycardia was compensated by an increased $A\text{-}V_{O_2}$ difference which resulted from both a higher arterial oxygen content and an increased peripheral oxygen extraction. They concluded that benefits with physical training in coronary patients at submaximal exercise levels result from enhanced arterial oxygen content and peripheral extraction, and, secondarily, from lower hemodynamic stress on the ischemic myocardium.

Thus, recent physiological studies suggest that much of the improvement in physical conditioning in patients with coronary

*Exercise and Coronary Heart Disease*

disease results from peripheral circulatory alterations, and that myocardial function itself may change very little. These studies suggest that this improvement in peripheral circulatory dynamics probably results in less stress on the myocardium which is especially beneficial in states of cardiac ischemia.

### Isometrics

Other recent investigations into the physiological aspects of exercise have involved studies of isometrics. Siegel *et al.*[32] studied six normal subjects, twenty-seven patients with coronary athero- sclerotic heart disease and six patients with idiopathic congestive cardiomyopathy. The method of study involved maximal isometric handgrip exercise. Results showed that isometric handgrip caused

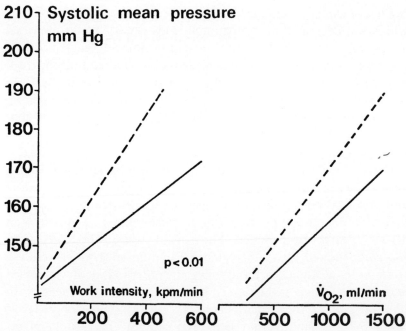

Figure   7.  Graph showing regression of the systolic mean pressure for leg exercise and arm exercise on external work performed and on pulmonary oxygen uptake. The interrupted lines represent arm exercise and the solid line represents *leg* exercise. (Copied with permission from Wahren and Bygdeman [34])

rapid and significant increases in systolic (22 to 39 mm Hg) and diastolic (27 to 36 mm Hg) blood pressure and heart rate (fifteen to twenty beats per minute). It was concluded that isometric handgrip exercise is a simple cardiovascular stress test which is applicable at the bedside, exerting its effect by increased blood pressure or afterload. Other observations [33] have concluded that such increases in pressure may be undesirable in patients with coronary artery disease or with borderline hemodynamic function.

Other investigation into types of exercises for coronary patients have included those involving the onset of angina pectoris in relation to circulatory adaption during arm and leg exercise. Wahren and Bygdeman [34] studied this in ten patients with signs of coronary artery disease. Both arm and leg exercise elicited angina pectoris in all patients. Anginal pain appeared at a smaller work load and a lower pulmonary oxygen uptake during arm exercise than during leg exercise and heart rate, peak systolic, diastolic mean, diastolic and mean arterial pressures all increased more steeply in relation to work load during arm exercise than during leg exercise. An example of this data is shown in Figure 7. This was attributed in part to the lower mechanical efficiency and higher sympathetic outflow during arm exercise. It was felt that these factors may reflect a larger component of static work with trunk muscles during arm exercise.

Therefore, it appears that different types of exercise elicit different responses from the heart and peripheral circulation. Evidence is suggestive of the fact that dynamic exercise, as opposed to isometric, is more efficient in conditioning the cardiovascular system and imposes less harmful stress on the myocardium, especially with regard to the increase in systemic blood pressure or afterload.

### Practical Application

In accord with such clinical and hemodynamic observations, leaders in exercise programming are being urged to design their training activities to deal with the simple factors of blood pressure and heart rate, that is to design training with the end point being to increase heart rate to a certain level in order to condition the heart. Dynamic exercises are preferred to those which involve

isometric maneuvers. Figure 8 shows examples of various heart
rates for given ages based on the data of Sheffield *et al.*[35] that are
currently in use in training programs. These rates are depicted
for the 70 and 85 percent of maximal heart rate (MHR) levels;
it is felt that the 70 percent MHR level is best used as an end
point for exercise, and the 80 percent MHR levels are best re-
served for an exercise testing end points in the presence of a
physician. Using these parameters through selected exercise over
a long period of training (such as a jogging), it has been shown
that a person can achieve a progressively greater level of exercise
with less acceleration of the heart rate,[36] thus reducing the work
of the heart for a given level of exercise. Likewise, through such
physical training, maximal blood pressure elevation can be decreased for the same level of exercise, again decreasing the work
of the heart. Therefore, with the more scientific approach to exercise, more benefits can be achieved with fewer complications—
complications that are frequently associated with inefficient efforts.

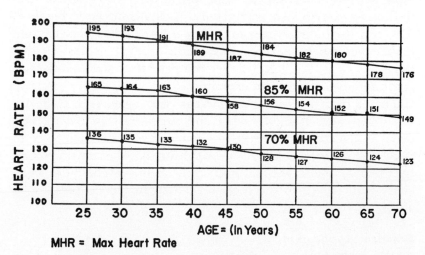

Figure  8. Graph showing various levels of heart rate in beats per minute
(BPM) expressed as maximum heart rate, 85 percent and 75 per-
cent of maximum. The heart rate is plotted with age in years.
The data is based on that of Sheffield et al.[25]

*Chapter III*

# SEDENTARY LIVING:

# A CORONARY RISK FACTOR?

INTEREST IN PHYSICAL activities and fitness in this country is not a recent phenomenon, for as noted in Chapter I, early leaders such as John Quincy Adams and Thomas Jefferson expressed strong opinions in favor of habitual exercise.

The past decade has witnessed the jogging craze, the bicycle boom and the resurgence of tennis. Mass participation sports continue to be popular the world over. In Sweden, 7,000 persons participate in the Vasaloppet cross-country ski race every March for little reward other than self-satisfaction and a cup of blueberry soup. Not to be outdone, three years ago the Danes started an eight-mile footrace around Eremitage Castle, the hunting ground of the royal family; the entry roll has increased seven-fold, matching that of the Vasaloppet. The Boston Marathon is in its seventy-fifth year, attracting over 1,300 runners in recent years on Patriots' Day.

In spite of the fads and the exercise extravaganzas, most citizens in the United States remain either apathetic, skeptical or confused. Perhaps the latter is related to medical warnings, early in the century, against the development of the "athlete's" heart. Neil Armstrong, whose very existence on the moon was so dependent on scientific precisions, once was quoted to the effect that he rarely exercised because man has only so many heart beats in a lifetime and he (Armstrong) didn't want to waste his. Satchel Paige, the legendary baseball pitcher, advised us to "keep the juices jangling" but to "avoid running at all times."

Amid the juxtaposition of exercise enthusiasm and indifference, wherein lie the facts relating to exercise and the heart? Perhaps the best approach is to first take a look at the animal experimental data pertaining to physical activity and training which has re-

17

cently been summarized so admirably by Froelicher.[37] In brief, the data can be analyzed under several categories.

## Animal Experimental Data

### Effect of Exercise on the Size of Heart Muscle Fibers

Multiple studies [37-40] confirm the fact that the animal heart responds to chronic exercise by enlarging. Wild animals, for instance, have larger heart:body ratios than do less active domestic animals.[41] An age factor seems to be important, however, in that while exercise induces cardiac hypertrophy in younger animals, there is actually a loss in cardiac size and weight in older animals.[42] While most feel that exercise-induced cardiac enlargement reflects hypertrophy of myocardial cells and fibers, several studies suggest that hyperplasia (an increased number of fibers) may also occur.[43]

### Effect of Exercise on the Coronary Arterial System

At least three types of investigations have dealt with enhancement of the coronary microcirculation following exercise training. Leon and Bloor [42] looked at the age factor in some detail and evaluated the exercise frequency factor in several groups of rats. The rats were divided into three age groups which corresponded to the human brackets of teens, twenty's to forty's, and fifty's to seventy's. Each age bracket contained a control group, a group that swam for one hour per day, and a group that swam for one hour two days per week. The results indicated increased capillary numbers, capillary:fiber ratios and coronary lumen areas in young adult rats, but not in their older counterparts.

Tomanek [43] ran a group of rats on a treadmill for forty minutes per day over a three-month period. He demonstrated an increased ratio of coronary microvessels to myocardial fibers, implying an enhanced blood supply to the heart muscle. He also noted that the greatest increase in capillary development occurred in the younger rats. Poupa [44] compared tame and wild rats and rabbits, finding a greater capillary network in the wild, more active animals. The capillary development was more impressive in younger animals, suggesting that these small vessels were more responsive to growth stimuli at an early age.

The above studies suggest that the microcirculation of cardiac muscle in animals will be significantly enhanced only if exercise is started in youth. The luminal area of the larger coronary arteries will enlarge in the teen group and in the young adults who exercise on a daily, rather than a twice-weekly basis.

The effect of exercise on the coronary *collateral circulation* of animals has likewise been evaluated by multiple research groups. The most widely quoted study of this type was performed by Dr. Richard Eckstein in 1957. Using a surgical technique, Eckstein narrowed the large coronary arteries in one hundred dogs. Those who developed signs of a myocardial infarction on subsequent electrocardiograms were divided into two groups. The dogs in group A were exercised on a treadmill for five hours per week over a one and one-half to two-month period. Dogs in group B were kept in small cages over a similar time period. The collateral circulation around the narrowed vessels was markedly enhanced in the exercise group as compared to the rest group. Cobb *et al.*[46] attempted to duplicate Eckstein's work by studying the collateral vessel development radiographically in fifty dogs, half of whom were in an exercise group and half in a control group. The former ran on a treadmill for forty minutes daily over a three-month period. When the coronary arteries in both groups were then injected with radiographic dye, there was no enhancement of collateral growth in the exercise group. One drawback to such a study, however, is that small collateral vessels cannot be demonstrated by angiographic technique. Burt and Jackson [47] were interested in seeing if an animal could develop the collateral vessels through exercise without first having had a large coronary artery partially occluded. Using a technique which was otherwise similar to Eckstein's, they were unable to demonstrate any exercise-induced collateralization, implying that one needed the ischemia of a narrowed vessel to stimulate the growth of the collateral vasculature. Kaplinsky *et al.*[48] studied the effects of total occlusion of a major coronary artery in forty dogs. Twenty-six of the dogs survived the insult and were subsequently equally divided into exercise and control groups. Coronary arteriograms were performed at the end of the study, the animals were sacrificed, and pathologic studies were then made of the coronary arteries. Both groups developed extensive networks of collateral vessels, but the exercise group had no better development than the control group. Perhaps if a vessel is suddenly totally occluded, as opposed to the partial occlusions induced by Eckstein, exercise does not enhance collateral formation.

The effect of exercise on the size of the *large coronary arteries* was studied by Tepperman *et al.*[49] and by Stevenson *et al.*[50] The former conducted a sophisticated experiment in which they compared two exercise groups of rats with two control groups. One exercise group ran a mile per day for thirty-six days while the other group swam for thirty minutes on a daily basis for ten weeks. The animals were sacrificed at the end of the study and vinyl acetate was injected into the coronary arteries. Potassium hydroxide was used to digest all of the heart tissue except for the coronary arteries, which were then weighed. Both exercise groups had significantly greater weights of the coronary arteries as compared to the control groups. Stevenson *et al.*[50] studied rats in a similar fashion, analyzing different frequencies and intensities of treadmill and swimming activities. He was able to show increases in coronary arterial tree sizes in all exercise groups as compared to nonexercise groups. However, in the strenuous swimming group, rats who swam for eight hours per week actually developed larger coronary artery diameters than those who swam sixteen hours per week. This study provides food for thought as the possibilities of a maximum exercise tolerance, beyond which no significant increases in the size of large coronary arteries accrue.

### Effect of Exercise on Myocardial Performance, Efficiency and Mitochondrial Morphology

Exercised rats, when compared to controls, are able to perform greater amounts of cardiac work and have an enhanced stroke volume.[51] When heart rates in both groups are artificially increased by cardiac pacing, the hearts of physically-trained rats were able to utilize more oxygen and produced less lactic acid than did the control hearts.

Holloszy[52] has described an increase in both size and number of skeletal muscle mitochondria after exercise training. In addition, there is a quantitative increase in the respiratory enzymes per gram of muscle tissue. The mitochondria of rat heart muscle were studied after various intensities of exercise.[53] While most of the exercised rats increased both size and number of myocardial mitochondria (similar to skeletal muscle), some mitochondrial degeneration occurred in the intensively exercised rats, suggesting that overexercise might have harmful effects. In another study digitalis seemed to prevent such degenerative changes.[54] Banister et al.[40] showed that the degeneration of mitochondria is more noticeable shortly after exhaustive exercise is begun and is much less once a training effect is achieved.

### Summary and Practical Application of Animal Studies

In taking an overview of the animal experimental data, several concepts are apparent. First, the evidence is overwhelming that exercise has a beneficial effect on the animal heart, be it an increase in the coronary macro or microcirculation, the mitochondria or in cardiac performance. Comparing young and old animals, it appears that exercise produces more impressive changes in the former. If we can extrapolate this to the human, one could build a case for developing exercise habits at an early age. The animal data also raises the question as to whether overexercise can actually be harmful. Again, putting this into human perspective, is the man who jogs twenty miles per week doing less for his heart than the man who jogs ten miles per week? From the available report on Clarence DeMar, who customarily ran over ten miles per day for many years, he did not show any cardiac deterioration (although electron-microscopy was not performed). Furthermore, treadmill studies in our laboratory on marathon runners, some of whom put in up to 150 miles of road work per week, show them to be in a much higher level of physical conditioning than the average jogger.

Let us turn now to the epidemiology studies in humans pertaining to physical activity levels and the incidence and prevalence of coronary heart disease. Excellent review articles have been written by Fox et al.[5] and by Froelicher et al.[55] The latter categorized the research into retrospective studies, prospective studies, autopsy evaluation and rehabilitation studies. This classification will be used below in a brief review.

## Epidemiology Studies in Man

*Retrospective Studies*

This type of study evaluates a group of persons after the development of coronary disease, seeking out factors in their past which might have predisposed them to the disease. One of the most often quoted studies of this nature is that of the London transport employees. Dr. Jerry Morris [56] conducted a review of the records of 31,000 men, ages thirty-five to sixty-four, and noted that the more sedentary busdrivers had an incidence of coronary disease 1.5 times that of the more active conductors who spent most of their day going up and down the steps of double-decked busses. Moreover, the sudden death rates and the death rates during the first two months after a myocardial infarction were twice as high in drivers. This study, though often the basis for the "hard sell" of exercise benefits, had certain significant weaknesses. For instance, there was no attempt to actually substantiate the activity differences between the two groups, nor was consideration given to off-the-job activities. Subsequent reviews of the data showed that the drivers had higher blood pressure and cholesterol levels than did the conductors, even when they first applied for the job.[57] Such differences could have made the drivers a higher risk for coronary disease for reasons other than the proposed difference in physical activity levels.

Dr. Henry Taylor from the University of Minnesota led a study on the mortality rates of white men employed by the United States Railroad Industry.[58] Death certificates for the years 1955 and 1956 were analyzed and they showed that the more active sectionmen had less than half the death rates from coronary disease that the sedentary clerks had. Thus, it could be surmised that men in sedentary occupations have more coronary disease than do those engaged in moderate to heavy physical activity. Further analysis of the data was rather interesting, however. Additional questioning of relatives and associates and detailed quantitations of on-the-job energy expenditure revealed that certain clerks actually expended as much caloric energy per day as did the presumably more active sectionmen. More significant was the discovery that men with coronary disease symptoms either retired or withdrew from the position of sectionman and entered into that of a sedentary clerk. The death rates could, therefore, be explained by a bias in job transfers and retirement tendencies rather than by any protective influence of exercise.[59]

Another interesting retrospective study was that of Frank *et al.*[60] who studied 55,000 men, ages twenty-five to sixty-four, who were enrolled in the Health Insurance Plan of New York. Over a sixteen-month period, 301 had experienced myocardial infarctions. Questionnaires and personal interviews with either the patient or his widow as to on-the-job and leisure time activity allowed classification into categories of light, moderate and heavy. The death rate following the infarction was 49 percent in the light group as opposed to only 13 percent in the heavy activity group. Thus, it would appear that even if physical activity did not prevent a coronary event, it might greatly enhance one's chances of survival. In a critique of the report, Keys indicated certain problems in its validity.[61] It seems that many of the men were ill prior to the infarction. It would be expected that the 22 percent with symptoms of coronary disease, the 19 percent with hypertension and the 10 percent with diabetes mellitus would be less active than the others, providing not only a statistical bias for inactivity, but also one for the severity of the infarction. Keys went on to re-emphasize prior observations that widows tend to underestimate the degree of physical activity of their deceased husband.

Dr. Curtis Hames, a private practitioner from Claxton, Georgia, had the foresight to arrange a coronary epidemiology study [62,63] in Evans County, Georgia, after observing that his black patients appeared to have much less coronary disease than the white patients, despite a greater tendency toward hypertension and high saturated fat dietary intake in the former. Analysis of the data confirmed the clinical suspicion that indeed black males had a much lower prevalence of coronary artery disease than the white males. After assessing the various risk factors through the use of the multiple logistics equation, Hames concluded that low social standards and relatively high physical activity habits appeared to account for at least some of the protective effect among the blacks.

A favorite subject for retrospective study has been the college athlete. Pomeroy and White [64] studied former Harvard football players and found no harmful cardiovascular effects from their prior strenuous activity. Indeed, those who continued to exercise in later life had fewer myocardial infarctions than the nonactive or formerly active groups. Prout [65] studied the records of 172 graduates of Harvard and Yale, each of whom had been members of the crew squad between the years 1882 and 1902. For each crew member, a classmate was picked at random to serve as a control. The life span of the combined crew members was 67.85 years, significantly greater ($p<.02$) than the average life span of the combined controls (61.55 years). When the cause of death prior to age sixty was known, however, there was not a significant difference as to the incidence of cerebrovascular and cardiac disease between the controls (seven instances) and the oarsmen (six instances). This study was somewhat limited by the inadequate listing of the cause of death in many instances. Schnohr [66] obtained information on 297 male athletic champions who were born in Denmark between 1880 and 1910 and compared their mortality with that of the general Danish male population. Although the causes of death were essentially the same among the athletes as among the general population, the mortality of the athletes was significantly lower under the age of fifty years. A recent study by Polednak [67] compared longevity and cardiovascular mortality among 681 former Harvard lettermen. Subdivision of the athletes by the type of sport revealed no significant differences in longevity. A unique finding was that men who earned three or more varsity letters had significantly higher coronary mortality rates than did the one to two-letter athletes. This data is again somewhat restricted in view of the inaccuracy of death certificate data and by the lack of follow-up knowledge as to exercise habits after graduation.

### Prospective Studies

In a prospective study, a population group is carefully evaluated and then closely followed for a period of time. Those persons developing coronary disease in the follow-up period are compared with those who are free of clinical disease, utilizing the initial screening data. The most widely-publicized prospective study in the medical literature is certainly the Framingham study headed by Dr. William Kannel.[68] Over 5,000 men and women, initially free of coronary disease, have been followed since 1949. While those with sedentary life habits had significantly more coronary disease than their less active counterparts, there are certain limitations to the analysis. For one, the level of physical activity was not precisely ascertained. For another, the physiological measurements (as level of obesity, vital capacity, hand grip strength, etc.) used to assess the degree of physical activity are somewhat arbitrary.

Paffenbarger [69] reported a sixteen-year follow-up study on San Francisco longshoremen. The study initially encompassed over 300 men, ages thirty-five to sixty-four years. It was possible to separate the workers into two levels of work activity, differing by over 900 calories in energy expenditure per day. During the follow-up period there were 291 deaths attributed to coronary disease. The less active group had a 33 percent higher coronary death rate than their more active colleagues. The differences due to activity were sustained even when blood pressure levels and smoking habits were taken into consideration. Unfortunately, serum cholesterol levels were not ascertained, leaving a big question mark as to whether or not this important risk factor could have accounted for the group differences.

The Seven Countries Study is an ongoing prospective study [70] involving a population of over 12,000 men, ages forty to fifty-nine, from the following countries: Japan, Greece, Yugoslavia, Italy, the Netherlands, Finland and the United States. When the data was tabulated at the five-year point, Japan had the lowest rate of coronary decrease while the United States and Finland had the highest rates. Physical activity levels could, perhaps, explain the low rate in the Japanese (who tend to be very active) and the high rates in the United States (noted for escalators and motor-driven bicycles), but certainly not the high rates in the Finns (the ultimate in physical fitness orientation). By using the multiple logistics equation, wherein all other measured factors were held constant while a single risk factor was being assessed, physical inactivity was considered a much less significant coronary risk factor than was hypertension and hypercholesterolemia.

The Goteborg, Sweden, study [71] is a fascinating project involving

834 men who were all born in the year 1913. In 1963, when the men were fifty years old, there were no clinical signs of coronary heart disease. Four years later, myocardial infarctions were diagnosed in twenty-three of the men, angina pectoris in eighteen men, and new electrocardiographic abnormalities were present in nine others. The incidence of myocardial infarction was significantly less in those whose occupations involved "heavy" physical activity than those in "medium" and "sedentary" job classifications. Unfortunately, leisure time activities were not considered in this study.

Exercise habits during leisure hours were, however, carefully reviewed in a recent publication by Morris *et al.*[72] Between 1968 and 1970 these investigators obtained weekend activity questionnaires on 16,882 men, ages forty to sixty-four. In the follow-up period to date, 232 of the men have developed clinical evidence of coronary disease. Each of the latter was matched with two colleagues who were not afflicted in terms of relative activity levels. Only 11 percent of the men who later developed coronary disease performed any vigorous weekend activity versus 26 percent of the control group. In other words, men who reported vigorous activity during the single two-day weekend assessed had about one-third the risk of developing coronary disease than the less active group. The shortcomings of this study were apparent to the authors, who correctly surmised that misclassifications could easily occur when assessing the activity of only a single weekend. For example, the active sportsman who was inactive that weekend because of an upper respiratory infection would be underscored, whereas the sedentary chap whose wife finally goaded him into a weekend project would be falsely classified in an upward fashion. Another deficit was that some of the forms of arduous exercise such as "vigorously getting about" are extremely difficult to determine, and more so to quantitate.

### Pathology Studies

Of the pathology studies, that of Morris and Crawford [73] has been widely cited. In the mid 1950's, these investigators performed autopsies on 3,800 men, ages forty-five to seventy, who died of noncoronary causes. The last occupation of the deceased was

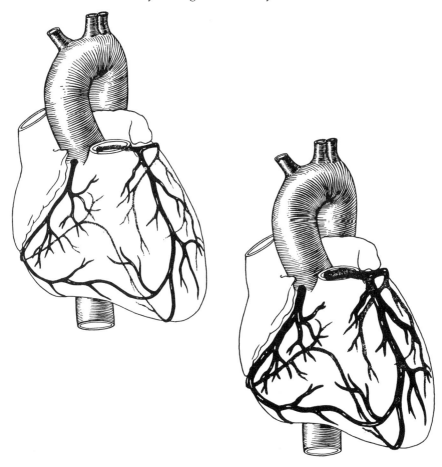

Figure 9. Autopsy study on Clarence DeMar, comparing his coronary vasculature (lower right) with that of a sedentary man of similar
age (upper left). (Artist's sketch.)

estimated as involving light, moderate or heavy physical exertion.
An independent assessment as to the degree of coronary atherosclerosis was made, and the results indicated that so-called "silent"
complete occlusions of a major coronary vessel (that is, a complete
occlusion without clinical awareness) were more common in those
of the light activity group. However, all occupational groups had
an equally high prevalence of less extensive coronary atherosclerosis, somewhat clouding the issue.

Another interesting autopsy study, previously alluded to, was that of Clarence DeMar.[12] DeMar was a remarkable man who competed in over 1,000 distance races over a sixty-year period. He competed in over one hundred marathon races, including thirty-four at Boston. His record of seven wins in the Boston marathon has never been equalled. When he died of metastatic bowel cancer at age seventy, his coronary arteries were found to be two to three times the diameter of the average man in his age category. Although he had some atherosclerosis, the overall vessel diameter was such that this was of little consequence (Fig. 9). While it is possible that Mr. DeMar inherited larger than average coronary vessels, there is nothing in his family history to suggest unusual physical development.

### Rehabilitation Studies

There are several rehabilitation studies [74-76] suggesting that exercise has a favorable influence on coronary disease. These will be reviewed in Chapter IX. Suffice it to say that such studies often have built in selection bias in that those without previous interest or experience in exercise will tend to drop out, as will those whose symptoms make them unable to tolerate the exercise program. The future looks promising regarding the acquisition of hard data in the field of postcoronary rehabilitation studies. The World Health Organization is conducting a randomized controlled study in European cities like Geneva, Switzerland, and Bordeaux, France. In the United States, the Department of Health, Education and Welfare is funding similar studies in at least four major medical centers. The project will be directed by Drs. Sam Fox and John Naughton. Georgia Baptist Hospital, via affiliation with Emory School of Medicine, will be actively engaged in this long-range (five to ten-year) study.

The multiple studies regarding exercise in the prevention of coronary disease in man are summarized in Table I. The trend of most studies is that physical inactivity may be a contributing factor toward the development of premature coronary disease. However, hard data is lacking to say unequivocally that physical inactivity is a major coronary risk factor. Hopefully, future studies will be devoid of the many weaknesses of previous reports. The

TABLE I

EPIDEMIOLOGY STUDIES: PHYSICAL ACTIVITY AND CORONARY HEART DISEASE (CHD)

| Type of Study | Major Author | Population Size | Occupation | Correlations of Physical Inactivity to CHD |
|---|---|---|---|---|
| *Retrospective* | | | | |
| London Transport | Morris | 31,000 | Drivers vs. conductors | Yes |
| North Dakota | Zukel[78] | 20,000 | Farmers vs. others | Yes |
| U.S. Railroad | Taylor | 100,000 | Switchmen vs. clerks | Yes |
| Evans Co. | Hames | 5,000 | Laborers vs. white collar | Yes |
| HIP of New York | Frank | 301 | Less active, intermediate, more active | Yes |
| Peoples Gas Co. | Stamler[79] | 1,500 | Blue collar vs. white collar | Yes |
| College Oarsmen | Prout | 172 | Athletes vs. nonathletes | No (but athletes lived longer) |
| Danish athletes | Schnohr | 307 | Athletes vs. nonathletes | No (but athletes lived longer) |
| Harvard football | Pomeroy | | Athletes vs. nonathletes | No CHD in athletes who kept active after graduation |
| Harvard athletes | Polednak | 681 | Athletes (1 or 2 letter) vs. Athletes (3 letters or more) | More CHD in lettermen with three letters or more |
| *Prospective* | | | | |
| San Francisco | Paffenbarger | 3,300 | Cargo workers vs. clerks | Yes |
| Framingham | Kannel | 5,000 | Active vs. sedentary | Yes |
| Seven Countries | Keys | 12,000 | Active vs. sedentary | No |
| Goteborg | Werko | 834 | Active vs. sedentary | Yes |
| British Civil Servants | Morris | 16,882 | Active vs. inactive (leisure time) | Yes |
| *Pathology* | | | | |
| England | Morris | 3,800 | Light, moderate, heavy | Yes |
| DeMar | White | 1 | Marathon runner | Enlarged diameter of coronary arteries |
| *Rehabilitation* | | | | |
| Israel | Gottheiner | 1,103 | Coronary patients | Positive trend |
| Case Western Reserve | Hellerstein | 100 | Coronary patients | Positive trend |
| Canada | Rechnitzer | 68 | Coronary patients | Positive trend |

"Seven Countries" study and the "Men Born in 1913" project (Goteborg) are in the final phases, and the end results are awaited with great interest.

The current shortcomings of our understanding as to the effects of exercise on coronary heart disease and upon longevity can be seen in the intriguing study by Dr. Alexander Leaf.[77] Dr. Leaf, while on sabbatical leave from Massachusetts General Hospital, traveled to Vilcabamba in the Ecuadorean Andes, Hunza, located in the Karakoren range of Kashmir, and Abkhazia in the Caucasus Mountains of Russia. These isolated areas were selected for study in view of their high incidence of centenarians per 100,000 population. While in the United States the incidence of centenarians is 3 per 100,000 people, the figure is 63 per 100,000 in Abkhazia. Dr. Leaf surmized that a low-caloric and low-fat diet, psychosocial factors and physical conditioning were among the possible secrets for such unusual longevity. Most of the centenarians continued to work and to exercise regularly at elevations of up to 6,000 feet, indicative of highly efficient cardiopulmonary function. Although once again "hard" clinical data is lacking in this study, it is of note that Dr. Leaf was so impressed by the effects of vigorous exercise in these people that he became a regular jogger upon returning to the United States.

*Chapter IV*

# EFFECT OF EXERCISE ON

# CORONARY RISK FACTORS

NUMEROUS STUDIES [80-84] have lead to the identification of multiple factors which seem to predispose one to premature coronary heart disease. A cross sampling of several such studies produces the following list of the more frequently implicated coronary risk factors:

1. Blood lipid abnormalities
2. Hypertension
3. Cigarette smoking
4. Carbohydrate intolerance
5. Physical inactivity
6. Overweight
7. Diet
8. Heredity
9. Personality and behavior patterns
10. Electrocardiographic abnormalities
11. Disorders in blood coagulation
12. Elevation in blood uric acid
13. Pulmonary function abnormalities

It has been difficult to assess the relative importance of a single factor in comparison to the others. Many of the factors are inter-related, such as blood lipid abnormalities, diabetes, heredity and obesity. Individual studies taken alone can contribute to this confusion. For example, compare the relative importance of diet and physical inactivity: Irish men residing in their native country consumed more calories and saturated fat than did their blood brothers residing in the United States; [85] yet, they had a significantly lower incidence of coronary heart disease. The latter was attributed by some to reflect their increased physical activity, which was mainly in the form of bicycle riding and manual labor.

Exercise might also be the reason why the Masai tribesmen of East Africa have such a low incidence of atherosclerosis despite eating foods extremely high in saturated fats.[86] It may also be the reason why farm laborers in Evans County, Georgia, have less coronary disease than their more affluent constituents, in spite of the fact that they consume more saturated fat.[87] On the other hand, certain studies have indicated that regular exercise is no panacea against premature coronary disease. The Rendille tribesmen of Africa exercise vigorously each day, walking upwards of twenty-five miles. However, they consume a diet high in saturated fat and have a high incidence of atherosclerosis, suggesting that diet is perhaps a more significant risk factor than physical activity.[88] An evaluation of risk factors in young persons with premature myocardial infarctions (prior to age thirty-nine) revealed that four men had exercised vigorously on a daily basis for up to three years prior to the attack.[89] One individual jogged from two to five miles per day. Another point against the importance of physical activity was a report comparing one hundred male military personnel (who survived a myocardial infarction at age forty or less) with a control group.[90] There was no significant difference in physical activity levels between the two groups. It should be pointed out that such reports can be misleading in that the accustomed degree of physical activity was determined by questionnaires rather than by direct interrogation.

Despite the deficiencies in the analysis of risk factors, they remain the most reliable simple screening device that we have available at present. Furthermore, the use of a multiple logistics equation has recently made it possible to assess the importance of a single risk factor while keeping the other factors constant. This sophisticated formula was used in the Seven Countries study, and when the five-year data on over 12,000 men was tabulated, hypertension, serum cholesterol and dietary levels of saturated fat seemed to be the most important factors, followed by cigarette smoking and physical inactivity.[91]

Coronary heart disease is, no doubt, multifactorial in etiology. Likewise, the effect of exercise is also multifactorial, inducing not only beneficial hemodynamic changes, but also interacting with the previously mentioned risk factors. It is therefore worthwhile to review the effect of exercise on the respective factors, for this might serve as an objective means of explaining the subjective improvements most physically fit persons profess. To do this let us take the thirteen risk factors listed at the beginning of the chapter on an individual basis.

## Blood Lipid Abnormalities

### *Cholesterol*

Lipoprotein electrophoresis techniques have enhanced our knowledge of the different types of hyperlipidemias.[92] Despite such techniques, the serum cholesterol and triglyceride levels remain the most practical screening tests.

Considerable data from numerous *animal studies* suggest that exercise has a beneficial effect in reducing serum and tissue cholesterol levels. Myasnikov [93] and Kobernick *et al.*[94] found that exercising rabbits had lower serum cholesterol levels and lesser degrees of coronary atherosclerosis than did the sedentary groups. In the latter study, thirty-six *rabbits* were placed on a cholesterol-rich diet for two months. Half were kept sedentary while the others exercised for ten minutes per day on a rotating drum device, a level of exercise which was sufficient to produce the cholesterol lowering effect. Several investigators have used *chickens* as their study model.[95] In general, the exercised birds (some of whom walked four miles per week) had reduced serum cholesterol levels and lesser degrees of large vessel atherosclerosis than did the matched controls. Gollnick [96] found that vigorous exercise could decrease the concentration of cholesterol in *rat* livers. Watt *et al.*[97] also studied rats and came up with several interesting observations. The rats were exercised on a motor-driven wheel over an eight-week period, and then underwent detraining over a similar time period. Training had a significant lowering effect on serum cholesterol, serum triglyceride and adipose triglyceride levels in the rats, but did not significantly affect the adipose levels in the heart or in skeletal muscle. The lowered lipid levels persisted during the eight-week detraining period, despite the fact that the body weight loss during training was regained.

In *humans,* decreases in serum cholesterol following an active physical conditioning program have been noted by many investigators. These include studies on prisoners,[98] air force officers,[99] postcoronary patients,[75,100] and the general population.[101] The latter study indicated that the amount of decrease was related to the percentage of exercise sessions attended over a six-month period. The duration of individual exercise sessions and of the total physical conditioning period was quite variable. Siegel *et al.*[25] reported a mean decrease in serum cholesterol from 247 to 210 mg% in nine blind men who were exercised for only twelve minutes, three times per week over a fifteen-week period. This was independent of any weight change. The latter is an important piece of information that too often is not referred to in reports of this nature. Campbell,[102] Berkson,[103] Mann [104] and Golding [105] reported similar weight-independent changes in other studies. The study of Golding was a longitudinal study and encompassed more than nine years of observations.

Numerous other studies have shown an exercise-related lowering of serum cholesterol levels and deserve mention. Johnson [106] found that eleven swimmers had significantly lower cholesterol levels during training than at other times. Karvonen [107] found that Finnish skiiers had lower cholesterol levels than did nonathletes. Chailly-Bert [108] studied middle-age men and found lower cholesterol levels in those who were more physically active. Three members of his sedentary group with hypercholesterolemia were exercised and experienced a significant lowering of serum cholesterol. Unlike the rat study of Watt *et al.*,[97] Rochelle [109] found that the decrease in human cholesterol levels during intensive physical training returned to pretraining levels within four weeks after the exercise regimen. Phillips [110] had a similar experience with six study patients. The serum cholesterol levels fell from an average of 298 mg% to 195 mg% during the eight weeks of running and handball activities, but rose to baseline levels during the detraining period (also eight weeks). When retrained, the levels fell as before.

The effect of exercise frequency, duration and intensity upon serum cholesterol levels has been studied in several centers. Daniel [111] divided male faculty members into control, mild, and moderate to heavy exercise groups. The exercise consisted of varying-speed treadmill work, five days per week, for seven weeks. While all three exercise groups had significantly lower cholesterol levels than the controls, there were no significant differences among the exercise groups themselves. Pollock [112] likewise found that there was no greater cholesterol-lowering effect in four exercise sessions per week than in two sessions. Konttinen [113] divided 187 Finnish military recruits into light and heavy exercise groups. Both showed significant decreases of serum cholesterol. Although the heavy exercise group did not have a greater decrease in serum cholesterol, they consumed more calories which added a confusing factor to the interpretation.

Few studies have dealt with exercise and serum cholesterol levels in women. Pohndorf [114] followed a married couple (both of whom were physicians) for a ten-week period during which both swam 1,000 yards daily. The husband then underwent periods of detraining and retraining while the wife kept active, though at a decreased frequency of exercise activity. Cholesterol levels decreased in both during training. The reduced level persisted in the woman despite less activity, but returned to the baseline level in the man during detraining. Metivier [115] compared the effects of stationary bicycle, vibrating table and free exercises in college women. Significant decreases in cholesterol levels occurred only with the latter type of exercise.

There have been many negative studies, including our own, regarding exercise and cholesterol levels. Despite sixteen hours of vigorous daily physical activity over a twenty-two week period, there was no significant decrease in the serum cholesterol of 101 marine trainees.[116] Holloszy *et al.*[117] studied twenty-seven subjects over a six-month period of vigorous training and found no change in serum cholesterol nor in serum phospholipids. Studies comparing cross-country skiers [118] and college athletes [117] with age-matched nonathletes detected no difference in cholesterol levels. Skinner [119] reported no significant decrease in the serum cholesterol levels of fourteen middle-aged men who exercised thirty minutes per session, five times weekly, for six months. Olson [120] randomly assigned thirty-one faculty members to sedentary and exercise groups. After a three-month period there was no significant difference in serum cholesterol levels between the two groups. The active group participated in "recreational" swimming, however, and one can question the intensity of such activity. Brumbach [121] divided college men into two groups of twenty each. The groups were matched for initial cholesterol levels, relative physical fitness, weight and age. The exercise group met three times weekly for ten weeks, participating in calisthenics, weight-lifting and running sessions. No significant cholesterol-lowering effect could be demonstrated in the latter group. Zauner and Swenson [122] trained ten middle-aged men over an eight-week period, using activities similar to Brumbach's. After fourteen days of training, significant reductions of serum cholesterol were demonstrated. As training continued, however, the cholesterol level drifted upward toward the initial values.

It appears then that there is no uniform agreement as to whether exercise *per se* has a significant effect on the serum cholesterol level. Many of the preceeding studies are difficult to interpret because true control groups were not mentioned, seasonal variations in lipid levels were not considered and details of concomitant weight and dietary alterations are lacking.[123,124] Furthermore, Mirkin [125] pointed out a marked fluctuation in serum cholesterol levels on a day-to-day basis during a long-distance running program.

### Triglycerides

In the well-controlled study of Holloszy *et al.*,[117] six months of physical training resulted in a significant decrease in serum triglycerides (from a mean of 208 mg% to a mean of 125 mg%) in fourteen men. This change was found to persist for only approximately two days following each exercise session, however. Oscai *et al.*[126] placed seven middle-aged hyperlipidemic men on a fixed diet and studied the effects of interrupted exercise sessions on serum triglyceride, serum cholesterol and lipoprotein electrophoretic measurements. The men covered three to four miles in forty minutes each day for four consecutive days and then rested from three to seven days. On the four exercise days the mean serum triglyceride level fell progressively from 235 mg% to 104 mg%. During the rest period the triglyceride levels gradually returned to the baseline level, taking up to seven days in some instances. The serum cholesterol levels were unaffected by exercise. The abnormal lipoprotein patterns of Type IV and Type V were normalized by exercise, but became abnormal again during the sedentary period.

Nikkila and Konttinen [127] studied two groups of Finnish army recruits. Both groups consumed high fat meals. One group marched for two hours while the other group was inactive. The serum triglyceride levels were significantly reduced in the marchers. Daniel [111] and Pollock [112] compared the frequency and intensity of exercise with the triglyceride-lowering effect. The former divided twenty-four male faculty members into four groups. One group remained inactive while the degree of activity was varied in the three exercise groups. All of the latter groups showed significant reductions in serum triglyceride levels as compared to the controls. The decreases were greater in the moderate and heavy work groups than in the mild work group. Pollock randomly assigned middle-aged persons into control and exercise groups. The latter were subdivided into two days/week and four days/ week exercise sessions. Both exercise groups had significant triglyceride-lowering effects from exercise as compared to the controls. However, those who exercised four days/week had no greater reductions than did the twice weekly exercise group. The usual postprandial increase in triglycerides was appreciably reduced by exercise in the group studied by Cohen *et al.*[128] Hoffman *et al.*[99] reported a triglyceride-lowering response to exercise, but furnished no information concerning weight change and comparison with a control group.

Several reports suggest either no change [129,117,130] or an increase in serum triglyceride levels following physical training.[101,116] This probably can be explained by an accompanying increase in food intake. Although Siegel *et al.*[25] found a mean decrease in serum triglyceride of 137 to 82 mg%, they did not feel this to be of significance. They made no mention as to how long postexercise the samples were collected.

The trend of most current studies suggests a transient lowering effect on postexercise and postprandial triglyceride levels. This might serve as an indicator for the frequency of exercise sessions (every forty-eight hours at least). The elevations in serum triglycerides during exercise training are most likely related to dietary alterations.

## Hypertension

Comparisons of resting blood pressures in active and inactive population groups have yielded varying results. Taylor [131] found lower systolic blood pressures in 416 active railroad switchmen as compared to 298 less active clerks. This difference was not present when the men were first hired for their respective jobs. No significant differences were apparent in the diastolic blood pressure recordings. Kang et al.[132] found similar results in Korean divers as compared to less active controls. Miall and Oldham [133] compared sixty heavy workers with 180 light workers and found that the former had significantly lower systolic and diastolic pressures. The differences could not be explained by social class standing. Karvonen et al.[134] showed that Finnish lumberjacks had lower systolic and diastolic blood pressures than did less active countrymen, and Morris,[135] likewise, had similar findings in comparing active and inactive London transportation workers. In the Seven Countries study [136] the more active men were not only leaner but also had lower systolic and diastolic blood pressures as compared to the less active men.

On the other hand, Chiang et al.[137] compared one hundred pedicabmen with 1,346 less active Chinese. Although the former were leaner, there were no blood pressure differences between the two groups. Similarly, no differences were shown between the blood pressure of active and less active YMCA members,[138] Chicago utility workers,[139] professional men [140] and civil servants.[141]

A drawback of many of the above studies is that total active hours (on the job and leisure time) are often not considered. Montoye et al.[142] took this into account in an assessment of habitual physical activity in 1,700 males over age sixteen years. The total energy expenditure was calculated from questionnaire interview data. The least active men had the highest systolic and diastolic blood pressures. This difference persisted even when the men were divided into specific age groups.

Considerable data has accumulated to indicate a modest blood pressure lowering effect of exercise both in normals [143] and in postcoronary patients.[75] Mann *et al.*[101] found a decrease in both systolic and diastolic levels after physical training, as did Boyer and Kasch.[144] In the latter study, the mean systolic blood pressure fell 13.5 mm Hg in twenty-three essential hypertensive patients who participated in a six-month exercise program. The mean diastolic pressure fell 11.8 mm Hg. Although the normotensive exercise group had no significant change in mean systolic blood pressure, there was a mean decrease of six mm Hg in the diastolic blood pressure. Mellerowicz [145] noted that trained sportsmen had an average systolic blood pressure of 20 mm Hg lower than the control group. Although Naughton *et al.*[146] and Clausen *et al.*[100] found a significant decrease in systolic blood pressure in nine cardiac patients who underwent four to six weeks of physical training, other investigators have reported no basic change in arterial pressure.[129,29,116]

The evidence to date suggests that exercise therapy can produce reductions in systolic and diastolic pressures in both hypertensive and normotensive persons. Similar changes probably occur in coronary patients, although additional data is needed.

### Cigarette Smoking

Fox and Skinner [5] indicated in a 1964 review that no adequate investigations have been conducted to determine whether physical exercise diminishes the desire for smoking. Such studies would indeed be difficult to substantiate as multiple variables are involved. For instance, all patients in our coronary rehabilitation program are strongly advised to give up cigarette smoking and are educated as to the deleterious effects of cigarettes on the cardiovascular system. Their response to such urging may be delayed and consequently falsely attributed to a subsequent exercise program.

One study that bears mention is the randomized evaluation of exercise training in coronary-prone Finnish males.[147] One hundred seventy-eight men were placed into two groups after matching for variable of serum cholesterol, age, systolic blood pressure, S-T segment depression in postexercise ECG, and smoking habits. One group remained as a control while the other engaged in physical training for an eighteen-month period. While psychological testing showed improvements in the exercise group, there were no definite differences with regard to changes in smoking habits. In another Finnish study, however, Kentala [148] found that regular attendance in a postinfarction exercise class was associated with an enhanced success rate in cessation of cigarette usage.

## Carbohydrate Intolerance

In 1924, Levine *et al.*[149] reported that physical exercise was usually accompanied by a fall in the blood sugar level. In 1945, Blotner noted improvement of glucose tolerance after exercise. Despite reports by Davidson *et al.*[151] that very intense physical training impairs glucose tolerance (based on only five subjects), clinical experience indicates that diabetic patients require less insulin when more physically active. However, well-controlled studies on physical training and insulin requirements are lacking. Nevertheless, Mann *et al.*[101] showed that fasting blood sugar level could be significantly decreased after a six-month exercise program (involving sixty-two men); however, the glucose tolerance did not change. There was no change in the fasting blood sugar level of exercising cardiac patients according to Frick and Katila,[29] but the group was small (seven men) and the frequency (three times per week) and duration of physical training (one to two months) was mild.

## Physical Inactivity—Overweight

Dr. Jean Mayer,[152] nutritional consultant to the President, has commented that the reason many people are obese is not because they always eat more, but because they often exercise less than nonobese persons. Nelson *et al.*[153] at the Mayo Clinic recently reported physiologic studies which indicated that one does not necessarily have to overeat to become obese, for as one ages, basal metabolic requirements decrease. If exercise habits remain the same or decrease in frequency, obesity can develop even if there is some reduction of food intake.

In comparisons of active and inactive population groups, the degree of body fatness is generally less in the former group. This pertains to London transportation workers,[135] middle-aged men in the Seven Countries study,[136] American railroad workers,[131] Chinese pedicabmen [137] and civil servants.[141]

Significant weight loss in normal and obese persons has been noted in response to prolonged physical training.[154,143,101,155,156] Analysis of studies reporting no change or a weight gain during exercise therapy frequently reveal appreciable increases in caloric intake.[157] Perhaps the most representative study is that by Mann *et al.*[101] wherein a small but significant weight loss and loss of subcutaneous fat was recorded in the exercise group but not in the controls or dropouts. It is important to note the effect of physical training on body composition rather than upon body weight. While the training experience might increase lean body mass, Boileau *et al.*[158] noted that the percentage of body weight as fat tends to decrease.

Regarding cardiac patients in exercise programs, Naughton et al.[146] found no weight change over an eight-month period of observation, although Hellerstein [75] recorded an average weight reduction of five pounds in a total of one hundred and fifty-eight men over a longer follow-up period (thirty-three months).

## Diet-Heredity-Personality and Behavior Patterns

Although exercise *per se* has no direct effect on the type of diet that is consumed or on hereditary factors, it has been shown to cause changes in personality and behavior patterns.[159] Most of the latter are subjective, however, although there are scattered reports containing more objective evaluations. Ismail and Trachtman [160] evaluated the effects of physical training on the personality traits on sixty middle-aged Purdue University faculty members, using the Cattell 16 Personality Factor Questionnaire. They found that the high fitness group were more imaginative, self-sufficient, emotionally mature and self-satisfied of conquering a certain goal.

In exercised cardiac patients, Hellerstein [161] was able to show a lessening of fatigue and an improvement in sleeping ability in addition to improvements in the depression scale on the Minnesota Multiphasic Personality Inventory (MMPI). Naughton et al.[162] found no significant change in the MMPI of a smaller group, but also noted the subjective improvements in sleep patterns and stress relationships. Hellerstein and Friedman [163,164] found that improved physical fitness had a favorable effect on sexual activity in post-coronary patients. An increase in sexual tension along with anxiety and alterations in sleep patterns was found in fourteen college students during a thirty day period of exercise deprivation.[165]

## Electrocardiographic Abnormalities

Electrocardiographic abnormalities, namely voltage criteria for left ventricular hypertrophy,[82] premature ventricular beats [166] and nonspecific T-wave changes [167] are additional coronary risk factors. Persons with left ventricular hypertrophy have an increased risk of death during an initial episode of myocardial infarction than do those without this finding.[168]

Strenuous physical activity may actually result in voltage criteria for left ventricular hypertrophy. Of twenty-one marathon runners studied, sixteen had voltage criteria suggesting this diagnosis.[169] While the hypertrophied ventricle of cardiac patients is felt to operate on the depressed Frank-Starling curve, this does not seem to apply to the hypertrophy of exercise.[170]

Hellerstein *et al.*[171] were able to show a disappearance of premature ventricular beats in four persons who underwent physical training. Blackburn *et al.*[172] noted similar lessening of ventricular ectopic activity after an exercise training regimen. Since ventricular ectopic activity may spontaneously subside, and since multiple factors can be operational, it is difficult to say with certainty that physical training alone was therapeutic. In the study by Pyorala *et al.*[147] (Finland), statistically significant increases in T-wave amplitudes were seen in the exercise group but not in the matched controls. It is doubtful that such a change has any impact on future coronary risk.

## Disorders in Blood Coagulation

In a review of the literature in 1962, Burt [172] noted a definite correlation between whole blood clotting time and occupational status. Those who performed more active physical work had the longest clotting times. He also noted that physical training could result in prolongation of both the prothrombin time and the blood clotting time. While ingestion of a meal high in fat tends to inhibit fibrinolysis and to accelerate clotting, these effects can be altered by postprandial exercise. MacDonald and Fullerton [173] studied a group of young men after breakfast of eggs, bacon and buttered toast. Provided they remained inactive, the blood collected three and one-half hours after breakfast clotted more rapidly than it did before breakfast. The enhanced clotting was not seen if the men went for a brisk walk after breakfast. Warnock *et al.*[174] walked chickens instead of men and found that those who walked four times per week had longer clotting times than did those who remained in cages.

Although unaccustomed strenous exercise can actually result in increased blood clotting and thrombus formation,[175,176] regular exercise, in general, will enhance fibrinolysis and, consequently, prolong blood clotting.[175,177,178] Forty-four college men [172] exercised on the treadmill until exhaustion. Eighty-nine percent showed acceleration of the blood clotting time and all displayed accelerated fibrinolytic activity. Astrup and Brakeman [179] have commented that increased blood fibrinolytic activity may be the explanation as to the beneficial effects of exercise in preventing thrombosis. They surmised that persons who failed to show this response to exercise training might be prone to coronary thrombosis.

Other risk factors can interact with the coagulation mechanism; for instance, several studies in addition to the one mentioned above have shown the accelerating effect on blood clotting by the development of hyperlipemia.[180,181] Such interactions need to be sorted out, and additional studies of a significant number of patients and controls are warranted to further assess the interesting relationship between exercise and coagulation.

## Elevation in Blood Uric Acid

Mann *et al.*[101] noted an increase in blood uric acid in exercising individuals. This may account for the cases of gout which developed for the first time in seven persons exercising under the supervision of Harris *et al.*,[143] Mann *et al.*[101] postulated that episode hyperlactemia might interfere with urate excretion.

Although Montoye *et al.*[182] found that high school athletes had significantly higher uric acid levels than nonathletes, these levels tended to decrease during the active season for the particular athlete. This suggested a possible beneficial effect of exercise. Bosco *et al.*[183] revealed that serum uric acid levels were reduced from 0.3 to 3.2 mg% in sixteen of twenty men who exercised over an eight-week period. The decrease was greatest in those with the highest initial serum uric acid levels and in those who underwent the most strenuous exercise. Calvy *et al.*[116] were unable to detect any significant changes in serum uric acid in marine corp recruits. More data is obviously needed to settle the relationship between exercise and serum uric acid levels.

## Pulmonary Function Abnormalities

A decreased vital capacity as a coronary risk factor was noted in the Framingham study.[184] Rechnitzer et al.[185] demonstrated an

TABLE II
EFFECTS OF EXERCISE ON CORONARY RISK FACTORS

| Risk Factor | Effect of Exercise |
| --- | --- |
| 1. Blood lipids | |
| a. Cholesterol | IE |
| b. Triglycerides | + |
| 2. Blood pressure | |
| a. Systolic | + |
| b. Diastolic | + |
| 3. Cigarette smoking | u |
| 4. Blood sugar | |
| a. Fasting blood sugar | + |
| b. Glucose tolerance test | NE |
| 5. Physical inactivity | + |
| 6. Overweight | + |
| 7. Diet | u |
| 8. Heredity | u |
| 9. Personality and behavior patterns | IE |
| 10. EKG abnormalities | |
| a. Premature ventricular contractions | + |
| b. Left ventricular hypertrophy | − |
| 11. Blood clotting | IE |
| 12. Blood uric acid | IE |
| 13. Pulmonary function | |
| a. Vital capacity | IE |
| b. Forced expiratory volume | IE |

+ = beneficial effects; u = unrelated; IE = insufficient evidence; NE = no effect; − = adverse effects.

average increase in vital capacity of 570 cc in four coronary patients who exercised over a twelve-week period. No changes in
vital capacity or in forced expiratory volumes were seen in sixteen
other postcoronary patients,[29,100] although the duration of physical
training was not as long (four to eight weeks). Exercise training
was recently reported as promising in patients with chronic obstructive pulmonary disease. Lefcoe and Peterson [186] summarized
four series, consisting of thirty-eight subjects. Beneficial effects
included significant increases in maximal oxygen uptake, ventilation and work load.

A summary of the present knowledge concerning the effects of
exercise on the coronary risk factors can be seen in Table II.
Beneficial effects are indicated with plus (+), adverse effects with
minus (−), and no effect with (NE). In other instances exercise
is either unrelated (u) to the factor or there is insufficient evidence (IE) to indicate a positive or negative effect.

*Chapter V*

# EXERCISE STRESS TESTING—A REVIEW

## HISTORICAL ASPECTS

FEIL AND SIEGEL [187] were perhaps the first to point out the electrocardiographic changes of exercise-induced angina. Their study was reported in 1928, fourteen years after Dr. Paul Dudley White brought the first electrocardiographic apparatus to this country from Europe. There was little enthusiasm for using exercise to evaluate cardiac performance until the following year (1929) when Master and Oppenheimer [188] described a "simple tolerance test for circulatory efficiency". This test, later to be known throughout the world as the Master 2-Step Test, paved the way for future studies and advances in the field of exercise testing. As early as 1932, Goldhammer and Scherf [189] were able to effectively induce electrocardiographic changes in over half of their patients with angina pectoris.

The past forty years have witnessed the evolution of exercise testing from the simple step test approach to some involving interrupted or continuous bicycle ergometry and treadmill activity. The former has achieved tremendous popularity in various parts of Europe, particularly in the Scandanavian countries. This has largely been attributed to the prolific work and writing of Astrand.[190] In the United States many medical centers are relying on treadmill testing with oxygen collection at the peak work load. The bicycle ergometer has been less popular, probably due to the fact that Americans are less accustomed to bicycle activity than their European counterparts. The advantages of the bicycle and the treadmill lie in the feasibility of greater work loads, constant electrocardiographic monitoring during and postexercise, and the collection of expired air to quantitate oxygen uptake and ventilation. The disadvantages include equipment costs and lack of a standardized exercise protocol, as many centers use their own regimen.

The reasons for stress-testing are multiple. Perhaps the main reason in the field of cardiology is the search for electrocardiographic signs of subtle coronary disease in the form of intra- and postexercise-induced S-T segment depression. One also looks for exercise-related cardiac rhythm disorders and the reproduction of chest symptoms during the stress of exercise, particularly those symptoms which are hard to assess by history alone. Still another reason for exercise testing is to quantitate the tolerance for exercise. At times it is difficult by history alone to judge a patient's ability to perform physical work. By directly observing the patient with valvular or other forms of heart disease on the bicycle or the treadmill one can get a better idea of his functional classification. Exercise testing also gives one a means of measuring the response to a certain type of therapy, be it in the form of a drug, an open-heart operation or an exercise program. The physiologist has long used exercise testing to quantitate the aerobic capacity of man by analysis of oxygen uptake during peak work loads. One of the first to do such studies using treadmill techniques was Edward Smith in the mid-1800's.[14]

## METHODS OF TESTING

### The Master 2-Step

What form of testing is applicable to the practicing physician? The *Master 2-Step* [191] is by far the simplest, cheapest and safest of all. For a patient with no cardiac symptoms, the presence of a physician in the exercise room itself is not necessary (although he should be within twenty feet of the exercise room). Cohen *et al.*[192] feel that this test is indicated in the initial evaluation of the patient. If the "augmented" test regimen (15 percent more steps than the basic two-step test) is negative or uninterpretable, one can then move on to bicycle or treadmill testing. Although the pulse rate during Master testing is said to reach 74 percent of the age-adjusted maximum rate, Cohen *et al.*[192] considered 20 percent of their tests on 305 patients "uninterpretable" because the pulse rates were less than 110 beats per minute.

Since time is a factor not only to the patient but also to the physician and the technician, a single initial test that is safe and vigorous enough is warranted. For this reason we prefer the treadmill. The variety of available testing protocols make it as applicable to the trained athlete as it is to the severely limited cardiac patient.

### Treadmill Testing: Georgia Baptist Hospital

At our hospital, we employ a regimen in which the speed is fixed at 2 MPH and the treadmill slope is increased 2½ percent every two and one-half minutes, starting from the level (Table III). We find the speed to be easily tolerated by most subjects and that there is less emotional overlay in testing if the speed is not progressively increased, along with the slope. Patients without definite cardiac disease are urged to walk to the point of heart rate elevation to approximately 85 percent of the normal maximal rate adjusted for the patient's age. Additional end points include severe fatigue or dyspnea, anginal pain, arrhythmias, S-T segment depression greater than 2.0 mm for duration of .08 seconds, or systolic blood pressure elevation to 240 mm Hg. A physician or physician's assistant and nurse, are in constant communication with the patient and the patient is urged to describe any functional and/or physical symptoms that develop as the testing progresses. At the end of the test, the patient is instructed to sit in a chair on the

TABLE III

GEORGIA BAPTIST PROTOCOL FOR TREADMILL STRESS TESTING

| Stage | Speed (mph) | Grade (%) | Duration (min) | Total Time Elapsed (min) |
|-------|-------------|-----------|----------------|--------------------------|
| 1 | 2 | 0 | 2.5 | 2.5 |
| 2 | 2 | 2.5 | 2.5 | 5.0 |
| 3 | 2 | 5.0 | 2.5 | 7.5 |
| 4 | 2 | 7.5 | 2.5 | 10.0 |
| 5 | 2 | 10.0 | 2.5 | 12.5 |
| 6 | 2 | 12.5 | 2.5 | 15.0 |
| 7 | 2 | 15.0 | 2.5 | 17.5 |
| 8 | 2 | 17.5 | 2.5 | 20.0 |
| 9 | 2 | 20.0 | 2.5 | 22.5 |
| 10 | 2 | 22.5 | 2.5 | 25.0 |

treadmill while immediate, one, two and three-minute postexercise blood pressure recordings and rhythm strips are made. If there are any symptoms or signs of near-syncope, dizziness or postural hypotension, the subject is placed in a supine position until stable. A direct current defibrillator as well as emergency cardiac drugs are available in the room.

Over the past eighteen months, two hundred-fifty patients have been evaluated by this method.[193] These include both outpatients and inpatients who were referred by their private physicians. Reasons for referral included chest discomfort (152 patients), clinical suspicion of ischemic heart disease based upon the presence of multiple coronary risk factors (forty-eight patients), abnormal electrocardiograms (twenty-three patients), history of arrhythmias (nine patients) and a variety of symptoms including dizziness, syncope and dyspnea (eighteen patients). The ages ranged from fourteen to seventy-five years, with the average age of 47.6 years. There were 176 male patients and seventy-four female patients. Six subjects were black. The range of test time duration was forty-five seconds to thirty-one minutes, the average being 14.3 minutes. The range of maximum heart rate attained was from eighty beats per minute to 180 beats per minute with an average for the entire group of 142.4 beats per minute.

Testing results revealed that twenty-seven of 250 patients (10.8 percent) had S-T segment depression of 0.5 mm or more and were considered to have abnormal results highly suggestive of, or compatible with ischemic heart disease. Thirty-two of 240 patients (12.8 percent) had the development of, or an increase in, premature ventricular beats, and twenty of 250 patients (8.0 percent) developed supraventricular arrhythmias (premature atrial beats, premature nodal beats or supraventricular tachycardia). Of this group of 250 patients, two (with histories of undocumented tachycardia) developed paroxysmal atrial tachycardia during exercise to document the arrhythmia; another, with a previous supraventricular tachycardia that required cardioversion, developed frequent premature nodal beats during exercise to further document a suspected abnormality to explain his tachyarrhythmia.

Further evaluation of the resting electrocardiogram in the 250 patients revealed that seventeen of the 176 male patients ((9.6

percent) and twenty-two of the seventy-five females (29.7 percent) had nonspecific S-T segment and T-wave abnormalities as interpreted by two independent electrocardiographers. This difference in incidence (increase in the females) is significant statistically at the $p<.01$ level of probability. Of these patients with abnormal resting electrocardiograms (S-T segment and T-wave variations) seventeen of twenty-two males (77.3 percent) and thirteen of seventeen females (22.7 percent) had positive ischemic changes on exercise testing compared to the male patients in whom only two of seventeen (11.8 percent) had positive ischemic changes with exercise testing. Of the twenty patients on digitalis therapy, three had positive tests for ischemic heart disease. (These three tests, however, had to be considered false positive because of the inherent difficulty in interpreting electrocardiograms when digitalis effect was present.) Of these three patients, however, two had classical symptoms of angina pectoris at the time of the ischemic electrocardiographic changes. Of the other seventeen patients on digitalis therapy, one developed ventricular premature beats with exercise; none of these had angina pectoris or electrocardiographic changes.

No one in the group developed hypertension (above 240 mm Hg systolic), syncope or extreme dizziness. No one fell, although one emotionally labile subject stepped off the treadmill unexpectedly. The postexercise recovery periods were uneventful.

Follow-up in this group of 250 patients was made by personal contact with the private physician and by reviewing their records

TABLE IV

FOLLOW-UP DATA ON 250 SUBJECTS UNDERGOING SUBMAXIMAL TREADMILL EXERCISE TESTING AT GEORGIA BAPTIST HOSPITAL

| *Reason for Referral* | Patients returning to increased activity | Patients with no change or decreased activity | Patients with no follow-up |
|---|---|---|---|
| Undiagnosed chest discomfort | 100 | 12 | 40 |
| High incidence of risk factors | 39 | 3 | 6 |
| Abnormal resting ECG | 4 | 1 | 18 |
| Syncope, dyspnea, dizziness | 6 | 4 | 8 |
| Arrhythmias | 7 | 1 | 1 |

for an eighteen-month period following exercise testing. These results are seen in Table IV. Of the 152 subjects referred for chest pain of undetermined cause, one hundred (65 percent) returned to work. Ten of these subjects returning to work or to a more active physical status had abnormal exertional responses suggestive of ischemic heart disease; of these, seven were treated with coronary vasodilators. Of the other fifty-two patients referred for undiagnosed chest discomfort, twelve had decreased activity and each of these twelve had abnormal tests for ischemic heart disease. Forty patients had no follow-up after eighteen months.

Of the fifty-two subjects in whom arrhythmias developed or increased during testing, only seven (13 percent) received specific treatment. However, all but three of the fifty-two returned to more activity with no clinical problems.

### The Bruce Method of Treadmill Testing

In the Preventive Cardiology Clinic, we employ the Bruce method [194] of multistage treadmill testing since we deal primarily with the cardiopulmonary fitness evaluation of young executives, airline pilots and amateur and professional athletes. The Bruce method (Table V) begins at a slope of 10 percent and a speed of 1.7 miles per hour. At three-minute intervals, the slope is increased by 2 percent increments and the speed by 0.8 to 0.9 mph increments. Few nonathletes progress beyond the fourth stage (twelve minutes).

Bruce and colleagues [195] have recently reported the results of the third annual test of maximal exercise in 186 middle-aged men

TABLE V
THE BRUCE PROTOCOL FOR TREADMILL STRESS TESTING

| Stage | Speed (mph) | Grade (%) | Duration (min) | Total Time Elapsed (min) |
|-------|-------------|-----------|----------------|--------------------------|
| 1 | 1.7 | 10 | 3 | 3 |
| 2 | 2.5 | 12 | 3 | 6 |
| 3 | 3.4 | 14 | 3 | 9 |
| 4 | 4.2 | 16 | 3 | 12 |
| 5 | 5.0 | 18 | 3 | 15 |
| 6 | 5.5 | 20 | 3 | 18 |
| 7 | 6.0 | 22 | 3 | 21 |

who were drawn from physical education classes, the Seattle YMCA and the Boeing Aircraft Company. One hundred and fifty-five men (83.4 percent) had negative electrocardiographic responses to exercise on three successive tests, using 1.0 mm of S-T segment depression as the criteria for any abnormal test. Ten men (5.3 percent) had three successive positive tests for ischemia. Of the remaining twenty-one men (11.3 percent), the results were variable. Seven with initially negative tests subsequently became positive on retesting. Six men were positive on two successive tests, only to become negative on the third. Seven men were negative on first testing, positive on the second testing, and reverted back to negative again on the third annual treadmill test. Such changes may represent reversibility of myocardial ischemia or random variations in the test procedure. Bruce found that interobserver differences in exercise electrocardiogram interpretation occurred in 5 percent of the tracings, adding another variable to contend with.

### The Spangler-Fox Method of Treadmill Testing

Spangler *et al.*[196] devised a treadmill exercise test protocol for screening high risk population groups. The test was devised with the goal of achieving near maximal heart rates without inducing physical exhaustion. The protocol involves alterations of both treadmill speed and slope, as seen in Table VI.

Three hundred and sixty-two asymptomatic men were tested by the above method after first having performed a double Master 2-Step Test. The men ranged in age from twenty-eight to sixty-six years with a mean age of forty-four years. Only three men were unable to complete the test because of fatigue. Three others were stopped because of positive S-T segment changes, eight because of frequent premature ventricular beats, and one because of paroxysmal atrial tachycardia. For men in the thirty to thirty-four-year-old age group, the mean peak heart rate was 167 beats per minute or 91 percent of the predicted maximum. For the fifty-five to fifty-nine-year-old age group, the mean peak heart rate during exercise was 162 beats per minute which was 99 percent of the predicted maximum. Five of the 362 men (1.3%) had unequivocally positive tests while eight others (2.2%) had border-

TABLE VI

THE SPANGLER-FOX PROTOCOL FOR TREADMILL STRESS TESTING

| Stage | Speed (mph) | Grade (%) | Duration (min) | Total Time Elapsed (min) |
|-------|------|------|------|------|
| 1 | 1.5 | 0 | 2 | 2 |
| 2 | 3.0 | 0 | 1 | 3 |
| 3 | 3.0 | 4 | 3 | 6 |
| 4 | 3.0 | 8 | 3 | 9 |
| 5 | 3.0 | 12 | 3 | 12 |
| 6 | 3.0 | 16 | 3 | 15 |

TABLE VII

THE ELLESTAD PROTOCOL FOR TREADMILL STRESS TESTING

| Stage | Speed (mph) | Grade (%) | Duration (min) | Total Time Elapsed (min) |
|-------|------|------|------|------|
| 1 | 1.7 | 10 | 3 | 3 |
| 2 | 3.0 | 10 | 2 | 5 |
| 3 | 4.0 | 10 | 2 | 7 |
| 4 | 5.0 | 10 | 3 | 10 |

line positive tests during or postexercise. Two of the men with positive exercise tests had normal postexercise tracings and would have been undiagnosed without the benefit of continuous electrocardiographic monitoring. The mean peak heart rate during Master 2-Step testing was 124 beats per minute, a rate achieved at the end of only the third stage of treadmill testing.

One advantage of the Spangler-Fox test is that patients could complete the six stages without having to jog, thereby causing less monitor-lead artifact from running movements.

### The Ellestad Method of Treadmill Testing

Using a fixed treadmill machine with variable speeds (Table VII), Ellestad and associates [197] have performed maximal stress tests on 4,028 patients.

No deaths occurred while testing by this method although there were two instances of nonfatal myocardial infarctions temporally related to the test and nine instances of transient ventricular tachycardia. Only one of the latter required specific therapy.

Criteria for a positive test for ischemia include:

1. An S-T segment depression 2 mm below the isoelectric line lasting at least 0.08 seconds from the J-point.
2. An upsloping S-T segment which is at least 2 mm below the isoelectric line at a point 0.08 seconds after the J-point.

Of 284 apparently normal executives who were tested on the treadmill, thirty (11 percent) had S-T segment changes of ischemia and ten (3 to 5 percent) had equivocal changes.

Of 236 other patients with positive exercise tests for ischemia, only 37 percent developed accompanying chest pain.

Advantages of this test over the Bruce method include simplicity and the fact that it takes less time. Patients have only one variable to contend with, that being the change in speed. A disadvantage is that the well-trained athlete will not be required to perform the high level of work which is demanded during the latter stages of the Bruce test.

The reproducibility of this test was impressive in a group of twenty-five men, ages forty to sixty-eight years, who were retested within one to ninety days. As regards treadmill duration time, 90 percent of the men finished the repeat test with less than one minute variation from the initial test. Twenty-two of the twenty-five men had clinical coronary heart disease and all had positive initial tests for ischemia. On the retest, 68 percent of the men developed ischemic S-T segment changes at the identical time interval as on the initial test, and 27 percent developed ischemic S-T segment changes within one minute of the initial test onset.

### The National Exercise Project Treadmill Test

Naughton, Fox and Hellerstein have recently devised a treadmill protocol (Table VIII) which is to be used in the HEW controlled exercise study on postmyocardial infarction patients. The protocol has one major advantage in that each stage of the test is one MET unit greater than the previous stage, allowing for easy conversion of treadmill work performance into MET unit values. Disadvantages include the lack of reported studies using this method for a busy clinic practice.

### Comparison of Step and Treadmill Energy Costs

Fox et al.[198] have published a chart comparing the approximate energy requirement of some step test and treadmill protocols.

TABLE VIII

THE NATIONAL EXERCISE PROJECT PROTOCOL FOR TREADMILL STRESS TESTING*

| Stage | Speed (mph) | Grade (%) | Duration (minutes) | MET (unit) | Physiological Functional Class |
|---|---|---|---|---|---|
| 1 | 2.0 | 0 | 3 | 2 | III |
| 2 | 2.0 | 3.5 | 3 | 3 | |
| 3 | 2.0 | 7.5 | 3 | 4 | II |
| 4 | 2.0 | 10.5 | 3 | 5 | |
| 5 | 2.0 | 14.0 | 3 | 6 | |
| 6 | 2.0 | 17.5 | 3 | 7 | I |
| 7 | 3.0 | 12.5 | 3 | 8 | |
| 8 | 3.0 | 15.0 | 3 | 9 | |
| 9 | 3.0 | 17.5 | 3 | 10 | |
| 10 | 3.0 | 10.4 | 3 | 11 | |

* Naughton, Hellerstein, Fox

Each stage of the various tests is quantitated as to estimated oxygen uptake and MET units of work. Clinical status and functional classifications are also provided. This chart is extremely useful in comparing results from laboratories who use different methods of testing. For those who cannot afford the luxury of oxygen analysis equipment, it provides a means of estimating the oxygen uptake for a given individual.

### Exercise Stress Testing Using the Bicycle Ergometer

The Europeans have long favored the bicycle ergometer as an instrument for evaluating physical work capacity. They cite certain advantages such as the low cost, lack of need of electrical power, and relative immobility of the chest and arms (permitting artifact-free exercise electrocardiograms). Astrand [199] notes that within certain limitations the mechanical efficiency of the ergometer is independent of body weight. Furthermore, he points out that the oxygen uptake can be predicted with greater accuracy than on any other type of exercise test.[200] A protocol for bicycle ergometric testing is shown in Table IX along with the predicted oxygen uptake for each stage. Women generally begin at a load of 300 kpm/minute while men begin at a setting of 600 kpm/minute. Each stage is six minutes long; at the end of each stage the work

TABLE IX

PROTOCOL FOR BICYCLE ERGOMETER TESTING

| Men | | | | Women | | | |
|---|---|---|---|---|---|---|---|
| Stage | Work load (kpm/min) | Time (min) | Predicted O₂ uptake (L/min) | Stage | Work load (kpm/min) | Time (min) | Predicted O₂ uptake (L/min) |
| 1 | 600 | 0–6 | 1.5 | 1 | 300 | 0–6 | 0.9 |
| 2 | 900 | 6–12 | 2.1 | 2 | 450 | 6–12 | 1.2 |
| 3 | 1200 | 12–18 | 2.8 | 3 | 600 | 12–18 | 1.5 |
| | | | | 4 | 750 | 18–24 | 1.8 |

kpm = kilopond meter

L/min = liters per minute

load is increased by 150 kpm/minute for the women and 300 kpm/minute for the men.

We prefer the treadmill device, particularly for maximal stress testing, since higher values of oxygen uptake can be achieved before leg fatigue and exhaustion set in. Americans are less familiar with bicycle riding than their European counterparts, and often have difficulty keeping up with the metronome. We have not had difficulty in obtaining optimal exercise electrocardiograms when proper attention is given to skin preparations and lead attachment. Moreover, we are impressed with the data of Bruce *et al.*[201] in which high correlations were shown between the duration of treadmill test time and the predicted oxygen uptake.

### Lead Systems

The lead systems used in most exercise testing centers are of three types: (1) Modified or conventional twelve lead systems. (2) Bipolar chest leads and (3) Vector (Frank) lead systems. Most bipolar systems, such as the one we use at Georgia Baptist Hospital, place the positive electrode at the V5 position. The negative electrode may be placed in variable sites. We prefer the V5R position, but others use the high anterior chest region or the right inferior scapular border. The latter is felt by some to offer a vertical component.

Mason *et al.*[202] use a lead system wherein the right arm electrode is placed in the right subclavicular area and the left leg electrode to the left midclavicular line halfway between the iliac spine and left costal margin. Hellerstein *et al.*[203] have used a system wherein the right arm electrode is placed on the forehead, the left arm electrode over the ensiform process, the left leg electrode at the V6 position, the chest lead at the V4 position, and the right leg at the V4R position. Redwood and Epstein [204] favor a lead system which combines a CM5 bipolar lead with a vertical lead (third electrode placed on the sacrum), feeling that inferior wall changes might be detected that otherwise would have been missed on the transverse lead alone.

### Target Heart Rates

For maximal treadmill testing we use the 90 percent of maximal target heart rate of Sheffield *et al.*[205] These values are compared with the Myrtle Beach guidelines [206] for age-adjusted target heart rates and aiming at 80 to 90 percent maximum aerobic effect (Table X).

In testing normal middle-age males, we do not find the Myrtle Beach target rates sufficiently stressful. Most patients in this category are able to progress an additional two to four minutes on the Bruce test before generalized fatigue comes on. By stopping the test at the target heart rate in these persons one would not get a true reading of oxygen uptake at maximum work. For this reason we prefer the 90 percent end points of Sheffield *et al.*[205] A reason

TABLE X

TARGET HEART RATES FOR EXERCISE STRESS TESTING

| Age | Sheffield Target Rates 90% of Maximal Heart Rate | Age | Myrtle Beach Target Rates 80 to 90% of Maximal Heart Rates |
|-----|------|------|------|
| 20 | 177 | 20–29 | 170 |
| 25 | 175 | 30–39 | 160 |
| 30 | 173 | 40–49 | 150 |
| 35 | 172 | 50–59 | 140 |
| 40 | 170 | | |
| 45 | 168 | | |
| 50 | 166 | | |
| 55 | 164 | | |
| 60 | 162 | | |
| 65 | 160 | | |
| 70 | 158 | | |
| 75 | 157 | | |

for pushing beyond the 85 percent maximum heart rate level in normal persons is evidenced by the recent report of Cumming.[207] Five hundred and ten men, forty to sixty-five years of age and having no evidence of underlying cardiovascular disease, were subjected to maximum stress testing on a bicycle ergometer. Criteria for a positive test included S-T segment depression of 1 mm or greater with a horizontal or down-sloping segment. For those with minor ST-T abnormalities at rest, a further S-T segment depression of at least 1.0 mm during or postexercise was considered a positive response, as was functional S-T segment depression of over 2.0 mm with the ascending slope being either 1.0 mm below the isoelectric point at the onset of the T-wave or having a rate of ascent less than 10 mm/sec. The yield of positive tests in the 510 men was sixty-three (12 percent). Of persons under age forty-five the yield was 4 percent, whereas it was 37 percent in those over age sixty years. Half of the abnormal responses developed after the exercise heart rate had exceeded 85 percent of the maximum heart rate. That is to say that had the test been stopped at the 85 percent maximum target rate, half of the abnormal responses would have been missed. This study, though provocative, needs documentation in other centers.

### Predictive Value of Exercise Testing

In 1931, Wood and Wolferth [208] suggested that electrocardiographic abnormalities which developed after exercise in patients with angina pectoris were an unfavorable omen. Thirty-one years later, Mattingly [209] reported the prognostic value of the Master 2-Step Test in 871 men, many of whom had symptoms suggestive of coronary heart disease. Of 145 with positive tests, 13.8 percent developed myocardial infarctions within the next three years and 38 percent did so within ten years. Of 726 men with negative Master tests, 1.2 percent developed myocardial infarctions within the next three years and 4.7 did so within ten years following the test.

At the Greenbrier Clinic, Brody [210] performed double Master tests on 756 business executives, ranging in age from twenty-three to seventy-four years (mean of fifty-four years). None of the men had a prior history or symptoms suggestive of coronary heart disease. Positive exercise tests (0.5 mm S-T segment depression) were recorded in twenty-three of the men (3%). Of the latter, 70 percent developed clinical coronary heart disease over a three to ten-year follow-up period.

Doyle and Kinch [211] performed a prospective epidemiological study with 2,437 men. Like the group above, none of the men had known coronary disease. A twenty-minute treadmill test was used in which the speed was fixed at 3 mph and the grade at 5 percent. The electrocardiogram was obtained immediately post-exercise and at the three-minute recovery period; no tracings were made during exercise. All tracings were interpreted by a single reader and subsequently reviewed in a blind fashion with repeatability of 96 percent. Seventy-five of the men (3.6%) had positive exercise tests. Over a five-year period of follow-up, 45 percent of this positive group developed other evidence of coronary disease such as angina pectoris or a myocardial infarction.

Bruce's group (Seattle) evaluated 186 healthy men with maximal treadmill stress tests. The interobserver variation in ECG reading among the four physicians conducting the study was 5 percent. Hence, the concurrence of ECG observations was 95 percent. Ten of 186 men (5.3%) had consistently positive tests on annual repeats. Twenty-one of the 186 men (11%) exhibited variable responses (thirteen with initially positive tests reverted to negative on retesting). In the three-year follow-up period, none of those with initially positive tests developed clinical evidence of coronary disease. However, at the five-year period, 13.6 percent of the initial positive responders developed such clinical evidence. Only 1 percent of those who initially had normal maximal tread-mill test developed clinical signs or symptoms of coronary heart disease. This study brings out two important points: (1) the use of a maximal stress test with electrocardiographic monitoring during as well as postexercise did not appreciably increase the yield of positive tests in normal middle-aged men (from 3 to 3.5 percent in Master 2-Step testing to 5.3 percent for the Bruce test). However, if one counts the patients in the Bruce study who were positive initially but were negative on retesting, the initial yield by this method would be 11 percent. (2) In view of the thirteen men who converted from a positive to a negative result on retesting this phenomena needs to be looked for in all future studies in which prognostic implications are made. In other words, the prognosis in those with variable test results needs to be compared with those who are either consistently negative or consistently positive.

Beard *et al.*[212] performed double Master 2-Step tests on 1,375 persons (1169 men and 206 women). Although none of the group had a classical history of angina pectoris, 42 percent had some form of nonspecific chest pain; hence, they cannot be considered as completely normal. One hundred and six of the total group (8%) had positive Master tests. During an average follow-up period of thirty months, 60 percent of the positive responders developed coronary heart disease by clinical criteria, 10 percent died and the remaining 30 percent were essentially well. Of the 1,269 persons (92%) with negative stress tests, only 2 percent developed coronary heart disease during the follow-up period and only 1 percent died.

Kattus *et al.*[213] studied 314 male insurance underwriters, some of whom had symptoms suggestive of ischemic heart disease. A near-maximal treadmill test was utilized. Thirty men (9.5%) had positive stress tests and the latter finding showed significant correlation with the serum cholesterol level and the nondiagnostic abnormalities on the resting electrocardiogram. There were no significant differences between the positive and negative treadmill responders regarding smoking habits, level of blood pressure, degree of physical inactivity, and family history of coronary disease. Over a 2.5-year follow-up period, three of the thirty positive responders developed a nonfatal myocardial infarction, angina pectoris or had significant abnormalities on coronary arteriography.

In the Seven Countries study, Blackburn *et al.*[214] reported post-step test electrocardiograms on 12,770 men, ages forty to fifty-nine years. Persons with ischemic S-T segment responses had a three-fold risk of developing manifest coronary heart disease within five years, even when other risk factors were held constant by means of the multiple logistics equation.

Robb and Marks [215] obtained Master 2-Step tests on 2,224 men, half of whom had a history of chest pain but only 3.6 percent of whom gave a classical story for angina pectoris. The age range was forty to sixty-five years. Thirteen and one-half percent of the men had positive electrocardiographic responses, (using the extreme criteria of 0.1 mm horizontal or down-sloping S-T segment depression, persisting for 0.08 seconds duration). In a follow-up period that extended to fifteen years and averaged 5.6 years, the mortality rate could be correlated to the degree of S-T segment depression as follows:

| ST Segment Depression | Mortality |
|---|---|
| 0.1—0.9 mm | ↑ 2.5 times |
| 1.0—1.9 mm | ↑ 3.7 times |
| ≥ 2.0 mm | ↑ 15.8 times |

Bellet et al.[216] performed double Master 2-Step tests of 795 male employees of the Bell Telephone Company. The age range was twenty-five to sixty-five years, and none of the men had evidence of coronary disease. Criteria for a positive test included either ischemic S-T segment depression of 1.0 mm or more or the development of multiple premature ventricular beats. Positive stress tests were noted in 11.9 percent of the men. During the three-year follow-up period, clinical coronary disease was diagnosed in thirteen of the ninety-five responders (13.7%) and in ten of the 700 negative responders (1.4%). Hence, the group of positive responders had an incidence of subsequent coronary symptoms more than ten times greater than the negative group.

Aronow[217] recently reported a thirty-month follow-up in one hundred normal subjects who underwent maximal treadmill stress testing and a double Master's step test. Using 1.0 mm of horizontal S-T segment depression or greater as a positive test, four of one hundred (4%) were considered to have abnormal Master's 2-Step test. These four plus nine others (thirteen of one hundred or 13%) had a positive ECG test for ischemia on treadmill testing. Of the thirteen positive treadmill responders, three (23.1%) developed other manifestations of coronary disease in the follow-up period. Of ninety-six persons with a normal double Masters test, three (3.1%) developed ischemic heart disease within thirty months. Only one of eighty-seven (1.1%) normal treadmill responders developed coronary disease within the thirty-month follow-up.

TABLE XI

PROGNOSTIC VALUE OF EXERCISE STRESS TESTING

| Author | Number | Follow-up (years) | Type of Test | % + Test | CHD Mortality | CHD Morbidity |
|--------|--------|-------------------|--------------|----------|---------------|---------------|
| Mattingly | 871 | 10 | Master | 2% (of 300) | ↑ 4.8x | 38% |
| *Brody | 756 | 3–10 | Master | 3% | | 70% |
| *Doyle | 2003 | 5 | Treadmill | 3.6% | | 45% |
| *Bruce | 186 | 5 | Treadmill | 5.3% | | 13.6% |
| Kattus | 314 | 2.5 | Treadmill | 9.5% | 10% | 23% |
| Beard | 1375 | 2.5 | Master | 8.0% | | 60% |
| *Blackburn | 12,770 | 5 | Step | | | ↑ 3.0x |
| Robb & Marks | 2224 | up to 15 (average 5.6) | Master | | ↑ 15.8x for 2mm ST dep. | |
| *Bellet | 795 | 3 | Master | 11.9% | | 13.7% |
| *Aronow | 100 | 2.5 | Master | 4% | | 25% |
| | | | Treadmill | 13% | | 23.1% |

*Denotes completely asymptomatic persons from a cardiovascular standpoint.

CHD = coronary heart disease

dep = depression

A summary of the prognostic value of exercise testing can be seen in Table XI.

### Sensitivity and Specificity of Exercise Testing

The true measure of any noninvasive study is how well it stands up against the most sensitive reference study, in this situation the invasive technique of coronary angiography. Before reviewing the literature dealing with this correlation, it is advisable to review two definitions:

$$\text{Sensitivity} = \frac{\text{True Positives}}{\text{True positives } + \text{ false negatives}}$$

$$\text{Specificity} = \frac{\text{True Negatives}}{\text{True negatives } + \text{ false positives}}$$

A *true positive* for our purpose is a patient who has both a positive ECG stress test and significant abnormalities on coronary angiography. A *false negative* is a patient who has a normal exercise stress test but an abnormal coronary angiogram. A *true negative* is one with no abnormalities in either stress testing or coronary angiography. On the other hand, a *false positive* is a patient with an abnormal stress test but a normal coronary angiogram.

For a noninvasive test to be highly useful, the sensitivity and specificity should both be as close to 100 percent as possible. Unfortunately, this is rarely possible and one is faced with using a specific test or a set of criteria by which the greatest number of "true positives" can be identified within a population without a high rate of "false positives".

With this in mind, let us review the available studies in which various types of stress tests (2-step, treadmill, bicycle) and diagnostic criteria (S-T segment depression of 0.5 mm, 1.0 mm, etc.) are compared with the findings on coronary arteriography. One must realize before doing so that the latter test is by no means infallible; when compared with postmortem examination of the coronary arteries, the arteriogram often underestimates the extent and degree of disease, particularly that involving the main left coronary artery, the proximal half of the left circumflex artery, and the intermediate portion of the right coronary artery.

Mason *et al.*[218] compared the results of exercise stress testing on an ergometer (bicycle or escalator) with the findings of coronary arteriography in eighty-four patients. The sensitivity (true positives) was 77 percent. In other words, of one hundred patients with significant obstructions on coronary arteriography, seventy-seven would be picked up on exercise testing and twenty-three would be missed. The specificity (true negatives) was 88 percent. Thus, for one hundred persons who had normal coronary arteriograms, eighty-eight likewise have normal tests while twelve would be given a false positive diagnosis of coronary disease.*

McConahay *et al.*[219] compared the Master 2-Step Test with coronary arteriography in one hundred patients who were evaluated at the Mayo Clinic. Using the criteria of 0.5 mm S-T segment depression as an abnormal exercise response, 63 percent of those with abnormal coronary arteriograms were detected on the step test. If the criteria of $\leq$ 1.0 S-T segment depression was employed, the sensitivity was reduced as only 35 percent of persons with abnormal coronary arteriograms were detected on the post-exercise electrocardiograms. Although there were no false positive responders (specificity of 100%) when the latter S-T segment criteria was used, the marked diminution in sensitivity offset this. McConahay collaborated with Martin in doing a similar study involving maximal treadmill testing.[220] Again, one hundred patients were evaluated. The criteria for a positive exercise test was $\leq$ 1.0 mm S-T segment depression (horizontal or down-sloping). The criteria for an abnormal coronary arteriogram was $\leq$ 50 percent obstruction of a major coronary vessel. The sensitivity was 62 percent, similar to the Master 2-Step data, while the specificity of 89 percent was 6 percent better than that of the step test (when $\leq$ 0.5 mm S-T segment criteria was used).

Lewis and Wilson[221] found that the treadmill test uncovered more coronary artery disease (as defined by angiography) than did the Master 2-Step Test. Using S-T segment criteria of 1.0 mm or more for both exercise tests, sixteen of twenty-six patients

---

* at least "false" in the sense that there was no large coronary vessel disease. This, of course, does not exclude small vessel disease and abnormal myocardial metabolic factors which perhaps could result in an abnormal electrocardiographic response to stress.

(61%) had positive double Masters' tests. The same sixteen patients plus an additional five (81% sensitivity) had positive treadmill tests.

Cohn *et al.*[192] favor the retention of the 2-step test as a screening procedure after validating it with coronary arteriography in 244 patients. They point out that the test is simple, inexpensive and safe, and, at the same time, provides a relatively high sensitivity rate (84%). It should be noted, however, that the false positive rate was relatively high (27%), thereby showing a specificity (true negative reading) of only 73 percent. Moreover, their original group was 305 patients, but sixty-one had "uninterpretable" postexercise electrocardiograms since the heart rates were less than 110 beats per minute. An S T segment depression of 2.0 mm had ominous implications in this study as 70 percent of these responders had three-vessel coronary disease.

McHenry *et al.*[222] quantitated the S-T segment response to treadmill exercise by digital computer in eighty-five patients. All patients had angina pectoris and were shown to have at least 75 percent obstruction of one or more major coronary arteries on cineangiography. A modified bipolar V5 lead system was used. The digital computer averaged the S-T segment responses of twenty-five consecutive beats from the immediate and the three-minute recovery periods. Seventy patients had an abnormal S-T segment response either during or post-exercise, a sensitivity of 82 percent. Twelve of the sixteen patients with a negative response had disease confined to a single vessel. Of the latter, the right coronary artery or the left circumflex vessel was involved in eleven of the twelve cases. In another group of eighty patients with chest pain and normal coronary arteriograms, the specificity was 95 percent (ie. there were 5 percent with a false positive S-T segment response to exercise testing).

Most *et al.*[223] evaluated the results of Master's 2-Step testing in sixty-five patients with angina pectoris and angiography-documented coronary atherosclerosis. The sensitivity was 58 percent, indicating that forty-two out of every one hundred patients with documented coronary disease would not be detected on the stress test. More disturbing was the finding that twelve of thirty-nine patients with widespread three-vessel disease had normal postexercise electrocardiograms. On the other hand, thirteen of the thirty-nine patients (33%) with three-vessel disease had at least 2.0 mm of S-T segment depression postexercise.

Roitman *et al.*[224] used maximal treadmill testing in forty-six patients with a sensitivity of 80 percent and a specificity of 87 percent. They concluded that if one could exclude a variety of clinical signs,** a normal maximal treadmill test will be associated with a false negativity of only 4 percent when compared with coronary angiography.

Although we generally reflect upon S-T segment depression during exercise, Fortuin and Friesinger [225] have recently called attention to the significance of exercise-induced S-T segment elevations. The patients were exercised on a stairway ergometer with constant electrocardiographic monitoring using a multiple lead system. Eight patients had S-T segment elevations during or postexercise in the anterior precordial leads. Coronary arteriography in these patients indicated complete or near complete occlusion of the left anterior descending vessel in seven of the eight cases. Four other patients developed S-T segment elevations in the inferior limb leads upon exercise testing. Each of the four was shown to have almost total occlusion of the right coronary artery on arteriography. Hence, it would appear from this small series that S-T segment elevation in the exercise electrocardiogram might predict the anatomic location of significant coronary disease with relatively high accuracy. More studies of this nature are needed to substantiate this.

There are at least thirteen studies to date in which an attempt to validate exercise testing with coronary arteriography has been made. Table XII lists pertinent details of each study, including the sensitivity and specificity values. The data can be broken down into each type of test, permitting one to compare the validity of one type of exercise test with another as follows:

| Type of Test | Number of Patients | Sensitivity | Specificity |
|---|---|---|---|
| Bicycle | 225 | 69% | 84% |
| 2-step | 652 | 68% | 79% |
| Treadmill | 259 | 74% | 90% |

** aortic and mitral valve disease, bundle branch block, hypertension, digitalis usage, LVH, and S-T segment abnormalities on the resting ECG.

TABLE XII
SENSITIVITY AND SPECIFICITY OF EXERCISE STRESS TESTING

| Author | No. Cases | Exercise Test | Criteria for + ET | Criteria for Abnormal Coronary Angiogram | Sensitivity | Specificity |
|---|---|---|---|---|---|---|
| Mason | 84 | Bicycle | 1.0 mm S-T dep. | $\geq$50% narrowing | 77% | 88% |
| Likoff | 74 | Bicycle | 1.0 mm S-T dep. | $\geq$50% narrowing | 58% | 68% |
| Martin and McConahay | 100 | Treadmill (maximal) | 1.0 mm S-T dep. | $\geq$50% narrowing | 62% | 89% |
| McHenry | 86 | Treadmill | 1.0 mm S-T dep. | $\geq$75% narrowing | 82% | Not Applicable |
| McConahay | 100 | Master 2-Step | a) 0.5 mm S-T dep. | $\geq$50% narrowing | 63% | 83% |
| | | | b) 1.0 mm S-T dep. | $\geq$50% narrowing | 35% | 100% |
| Fitzgibbon | 87 | Master 2-Step | 0.5 mm S-T dep. | Special index (approximately 50% obstruction) | 67% | 84% |
| Lewis | 26 | a) Master 2-Step | 1.0 mm S-T dep. | | 61% | 91% |
| | | b) Treadmill (Bruce) | | | 81% | 100% |
| Roitman | 46 | Treadmill (maximal) | 1.0 mm S-T dep. | $\geq$50% narrowing | 80% | 87% |
| Most | 65 | Master 2-Step | 1.0 mm S-T dep. | $\geq$50% narrowing | 58% | Not Applicable |
| Cohn | 244 | Master 2-Step | 0.5 mm S-T dep. | $\geq$50% narrowing | 84% | 73% |
| Kassebaum | 67 | Bicycle | 0.5 mm S-T dep. | $\geq$50% narrowing | 73% | 97% |
| | | | 1.0 mm S-T dep. | | 71% | 97% |
| Demany | 75 | Master 2-Step | 1.0 mm S-T dep. | $\geq$50% narrowing | 43% | 69% |
| Hultgren | 55 | Master 2-Step | 1.0 mm S-T dep. | $\geq$50% narrowing | 60% | 100% |

ET = exercise test

The treadmill method scores the highest in validity, with a false positive rate of 10 percent (versus 21 percent for the Master's test). The false negative rates for all the test methods (26 to 32%) is sizeable and accounts for the continued striving to enhance the yield of exercise testing in coronary heart disease.

### Recent Advances in Stress Testing

While future modifications are likely in the selection of test protocols and in the electrocardiographic criteria utilized, it might be that ancillary noninvasive techniques will be required to supplement the exercise test in hopes of enhancing the sensitivity. One such ancillary technique is that of recording the *systolic time intervals* pre- and postexercise. By simultaneously recording the carotid pulse, the electrocardiogram and the phonocardiogram, one can derive the left ventricular ejection time (LVET) the $Q-S_2$ interval, and the pre-ejection period (PEP). Weissler et al.[226] have recently emphasized the use of these measurements to appraise ventricular performance. As left ventricular performance decreased, characteristic changes are noted in the rate-corrected systolic time intervals. The PEP, an index of the rate of rise of the left ventricular pressure plus electromechanical delay, is shown to lengthen, while the LVET tends to shorten in patients with left ventricular dysfunction. The result is a significant increase in the PEP/LVET ratio. Hemodynamic studies have shown a close correlation between this ratio and measured cardiac index and stroke volume index.[227] Inotropic influences, such as digitalis administration, tend to shorten both the PEP and the LVET, thereby shortening the overall measurement of electromechanical systole $(Q-S_2)$.

Pouget *et al.*[228] made comparisons between twenty normals and twenty patients with angina pectoris, matching the groups according to age. The angina patients had a slightly longer PEP and a shorter LVET at rest but the overlap was considerable between the patients and the normal controls. Repeat measurements of the systolic time intervals after two to four-minute exercise sessions tended to separate the two groups. The normals showed a slight shortening of the PEP and LVET postexercise. The angina patients shortened their PEP and lengthened their LVET. The latter, a seemingly paradoxical response, may have been due to the inability of the Frank-Starling mechanism and catecholamine-mediated increased contractility to offset the delay in LVET induced by the temporary decrease in left ventricular performance associated with exercise.

Whitsett and Naughton [229] studied four groups of individuals (sedentary healthy, active healthy, postmyocardial infarction sedentary and postmyocardial infarction reconditioned). In the postinfarction inactive group, the LVET lengthened after treadmill testing, comparable to the data of Pouget *et al.* In the coronary active group (conditioned) the LVET was significantly shortened, suggesting an improvement in left ventricular performance due to physical training.

McConahay *et al.*[230] compared resting and postexercise systolic time intervals in thirty-three normal subjects and thirty-two age and sex-matched patients with coronary heart disease. At rest, the coronary group showed a longer rate-corrected PEP, a shorter rate-corrected LVET, and a larger PEP/LVET ratio than the normals with significance at the P<.01 level. Postexercise values showed the same significant difference. Both groups (normals and coronary patients) had significant decreases in the rate-corrected PEP, increases in the LVET and lessening of the PEP/LVET ratio postexercise.

Gilbert and Cantwell [231] studied twenty-nine normal sedentary persons, thirteen normal trained persons and twenty-one persons with well-documented coronary heart disease. The data from this study was in accord with previous investigators showing the postexercise increase in LVET in coronary patients. The postexercise LVET seemed of value as another objective means of assessing the physical training effect. Although there were no significant differences at rest between the rate-corrected LVET of normal sedentary and normal trained persons, significant differences (P<.05) did develop on the two-minute postexercise tracings. As previously mentioned in another study, the postexercise shortening of the LVET might also be useful in determining a similar training effect in coronary patients who are engaged in physical training programs.

A brief summary of the systolic time interval data is noted in Table XIII.[3]

TABLE XIII

SYSTOLIC TIME INTERVALS AFTER EXERCISE STRESS TESTING

| Pouget, et al. | PEP after acute exercise | LVET after acute exercise |
|---|:---:|:---:|
| Normals | ↓ | ↓ |
| Angina patients | ↓ ↓ | ↑ |
| *Whitsett and Naughton* | | |
| Normals (inactive) | ↓ | sl ↓ |
| Normals (active) | ↓ | ↓ |
| Coronary patients (inactive) | ↓ ↓ | sl ↑ |
| Coronary patients (active) | ↓ ↓ | ↓ |
| *Gilbert and Cantwell* | | |
| Normal (inactive) | ↓ | ↓ |
| Normal (active) | ↓ | ↓ ↓ |
| Coronary patients (inactive) | ↓ | ↑ |

PEP = pre-ejection period
LVET = left ventricular ejection time
sl = slightly

Another noninvasive technique which has been utilized in conjunction with exercise stress testing, is *phono and apex-cardiography*. Benchimol and Dimond [232] were among the first to study the effect of Master's 2-Step exercise on the latter in normal subjects and in patients with coronary heart disease. They found that the a-wave ratio (a/e-o) was significantly greater in the coronary patients. Aronow *et al.*[233] found significant differences in the postexercise a-wave ratios between normal subjects who had an abnormal maximal treadmill test and normal subjects who had a normal treadmill test. The postexercise a-wave ratio was 19.7 percent in the former and 12.8 percent in the latter, the significance being at the $P<.001$ level. Over half of the so-called normals with abnormal treadmill tests had postexercise a-wave ratios of 20 percent as compared to only 9 percent of the normal subjects with normal treadmill tests. The mechanism behind the augmented a-wave is probably related to the increased resistance of a left ventricle that becomes ischemic during or postexercise. Because of the added resistance, the left ventricular end-diastolic pressure rises, necessitating a more vigorous left atrial contraction to achieve adequate ventricular filling.

Aronow *et al.*[233] also compared resting and postexercise (Master 2-Step) phonocardiograms in one hundred normal subjects and one hundred patients with angina pectoris. On the resting recording, fourth heart sounds were present in 14 percent of the normals and in 43 percent of the coronary patients. After exercise, 94 percent of the patients and 29 percent of the normals had fourth heart sounds. Third heart sounds were recorded at rest in 1 percent of the normals and in 15 percent of the angina patients. Following exercise testing, 60 percent of the angina patients had third heart sounds, versus 11 percent of the normals. Of the eleven normal subjects who developed third heart sounds post-double Master's test, four (36%) had abnormal maximal treadmill stress tests and seven (64%) had normal treadmill responses. The incidence of both third and fourth heart sounds was significantly greater in the normal subjects having abnormal maximal treadmill stress tests than in the normal subjects who had normal treadmill tests.

A noninvasive technique that has stimulated great interest within the past few years is *echocardiography*. This technique of cardiac examination by reflected ultrasound was first introduced in 1954. Although there are no reports on pre- and postexercise echocardiograms, there may be some merit in looking into this for the following reason: By using ultrasound to measure the distance between the interventricular septum and an area of the posterior left ventricular wall, one can assess the left ventricular systolic and diastolic volumes.[234] With the former figures, the stroke volume and ejection fraction can be estimated with reasonable accuracy. A measure of stroke volume change after treadmill, bicycle or step testing could be an important clue to cardiac function in normal subjects and in coronary patients, both trained and untrained.

Zaret *et al.*[235] recently described the use of radioactive potassium injections followed by myocardial perfusion scanning both pre-

and postexercise. Sixteen of nineteen patients with angina pectoris showed regions of decreased $^{43}K$ accumulations during exercise that were not present at rest. The zones of decreased radioactivity corresponded to abnormalities noted at coronary arteriography.

### Exercise Testing for Evaluation and Detection of Cardiac Rhythm Disturbances

In addition to its use in detecting repolarization abnormalities, exercise stress testing is also of diagnostic aid in assessing cardiac rhythm and conduction disturbances. The arrhythmia-prone person can sometimes be spotted on submaximal or maximal exercise testing. In addition, the stability and significance of a rhythm disorder can sometimes be demonstrated by this method. An example of the latter is as follows:

> A fifty-two-year-old woman was referred to a cardiologist because of a history of palpitations which dated back twenty years or more. The cardiopulmonary examination was normal. The resting electrocardiogram was unremarkable except for frequent premature ventricular beats (Fig. 10), at times occurring in trigeminy. The patient underwent treadmill testing by the Bruce method, attaining a maximal heart rate of 167 beats per minute. As soon as the heart rate exceeded a rate of eighty/minute, the patient had no further premature beats (Fig. 11). There were no ischemic changes on the electrocardiogram during or after exercise.

The normal response to maximal exercise and the complete cessation of ventricular ectopic beats made it highly likely that the ventricular ectopy at rest was of a relatively benign nature, even though recent findings may question the "benign" nature of exercise-related cessation of ectopic beats.[236]

Gooch [237] has perhaps the most extensive experience of anyone in this field, having performed exercise tests to record changes in rhythm and conduction in over 3000 subjects over a five-year period. His findings can be summarized as follows:

1. Premature ventricular beats occur frequently during exercise stress testing and do not by themselves necessarily indicate underlying cardiac disease unless they occur in bigeminy or in paroxysms of multifocal ventricular beats.

2. Atrial arrhythmias are fairly common after exercise, occurring both in normal subjects and in those with known cardiac disease.

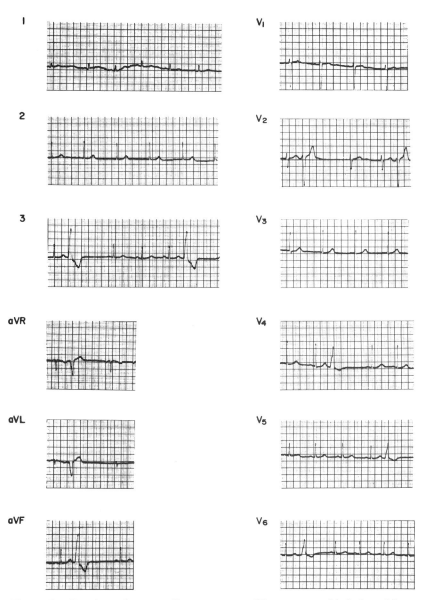

Figure 10. Resting electrocardiogram on a fifty-two-year-old lady with a chronic history of frequent ventricular premature beats.

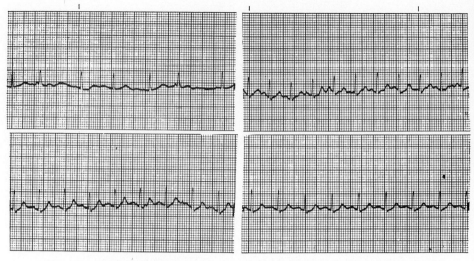

Figure 11. Suppression of ventricular premature beats during exercise in the patient described in Figure 10. Upper left tracing shows the ventricular premature beats at rest. There is suppression during exercise (upper right), immediately postexercise (lower left) and two minutes postexercise (lower right).

Brief paroxysms of supraventricular tachyarrhythmias are not unusual during exercise.

3. Exercise testing might be of help in identifying the inadequately-digitalized patient with atrial fibrillation (who will develop enhanced A-V conduction). On the other hand, rhythm suggesting digitalis intoxication can sometimes be brought out by exercise stress testing.

4. Complete bundle branch block (left or right) can be induced by exercise, most likely as a result of the "critical rate" phenomenon.

5. If A-V block is present on the resting electrocardiogram it is difficult to predict the response to exercise (ie. the condition may either improve, stay the same or worsen).

Exercise stress testing has been of value in separating the patient with congenital complete heart block from the one with acquired complete heart block. The ventricular rate of the former usually increases significantly during exercise, while that of the latter often shows very little rate increase.

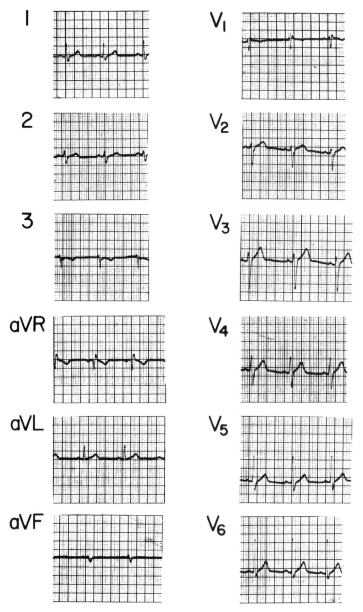

Figure 12. Resting electrocardiogram on a thirty-two-year-old physician and distance runner, showing left anterior hemiblock and incomplete right bundle branch block.

BASELINE TRACING                                              DURING EXERCISE

IMMEDIATE POST EXERCISE                                      2 MINUTE POST EXERCISE

5 MINUTE POST EXERCISE

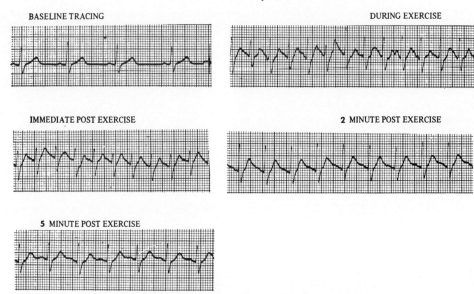

Figure 13. Exercise electrocardiogram of the subject in Figure 12.

An example of the use of treadmill testing to assess the significance of recently acquired bifascicular conduction disturbances is seen below:

> A thirty-two-year-old very athletic physician was seen by one of the authors (JDC) in consultation. Over a five-year period he had developed left anterior hemiblock and incomplete right bundle branch block (Fig. 12). The patient advanced to the fifth stage of the Bruce treadmill test with no evidence of myocardial ischemia and no increase in the degree of block (Fig. 13). His oxygen uptake was 55 ml/kg/minute, placing him in the very high category for his group. He was advised to continue his active ways and to undergo resting and exercise electrocardiography at six to twelve-month intervals.

Vedin *et al.*[238] correlated exercise-induced ventricular ectopic beats to several coronary risk factors (elevated blood pressure and fasting blood glucose, cardiac enlargement on x-ray, ischemic exercise electrocardiogram changes) in the Goteborg study of men born in 1913. Two of the men who had frequent ventricular premature beats precipitated by exercise died suddenly and unexpectedly, raising the possibility that this finding might be an important predictor of high risk for future sudden death.

Exercise stress testing has been of help in evaluating patients with pacemakers. Singer *et al.*[239] discovered various types of arrhythmias in 75 percent of twenty-seven patients with permanent pacemakers, including five instances of ventricular tachycardia. As patients developed new rhythms during testing it became possible to assess the type of pacemaker (fixed-rate or demand) and how well the sensing mechanism of the latter was functioning.

### Miscellaneous Aspects of Exercise Testing

Exercise testing is highly adaptable and extremely flexible. It may be used to evaluate peripheral vascular insufficiency [240] or to help in the assessment of a new surgical procedure such as aorto-coronary saphenous vein graft operations.[241] An arm ergometer test may be employed in amputees.[242] Patients with Prinzmetal (or "variant") angina may need to start at higher initial work loads as the warm-up phenomenon may obscure the electrocardiographic findings.[243]

Caution should be used in avoiding the overinterpretation of the exercise electrocardiogram. Murray [244] will consider an exer-

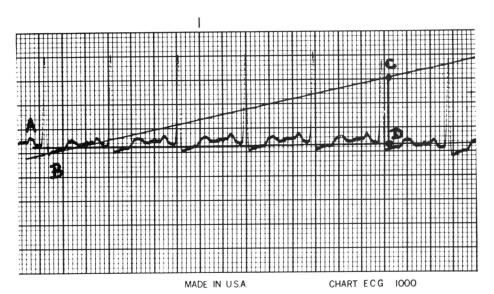

MADE IN U.S.A.             CHART ECG  1000

Figure 14.  Calculation of the S-T segment slope of the exercise electrocardio-gram in Figure 12.

cise electrocardiogram positive, based on the magnitude of S-T segment junctional depression alone. If the S-T (J) depression is 1.0 mm or greater, the S-T slope (mv/sec.) is subtracted from it. If the result is less than zero, the test is considered abnormal. The S-T slope is calculated (Fig. 14) by drawing a line along the S-T segment and extending it to a point three seconds distal on the electrocardiogram paper (point D). The distance from point D to the isoelectric line (point C) is the S-T slope. Although such additional calculations might increase the sensitivity of exercise testing, this remains to be proven. Moreover, long-term follow-up data on patients with junctional S-T segment changes alone is lacking. Recent studies suggest that false positive readings may be commonplace in the presence of left ventricular hypertrophy.[245] They may also be noted after glucose ingestion.[246]

### Summary

A brief historical review of exercise stress testing has been presented. The various methods of testing are described, including specific test protocols, lead systems, target heart rates and criteria for positive tests. The predictive value of exercise testing, along with the sensitivity and specificity of such testing, is reviewed in detail. A discussion of noninvasive measures which may complement exercise stress testing (such as systolic time intervals, apex and phonocardiography, and echocardiography) is provided. The use of exercise testing to assess cardiac rhythm and conduction is reviewed. It would appear that exercise stress testing plays a significant role in our armamentarium against coronary heart disease. In spite of obvious limitations, such as false negative readings of 25 percent and an inability to predict the extent and locations of coronary disease,[247] it is a safe, simple and relatively inexpensive way to quantitate cardiovascular performance and to detect subclinical coronary disease or tendencies for such.

*Chapter VI*

# GUIDELINES TO

# EXERCISE TRAINING

P RIOR TO COMMENCING any physical conditioning program, it is absolutely essential that certain medical requirements be met.[248] The *apparently healthy person* under age thirty years needs only to have a complete medical history and physical examination within the preceding year. For those *between ages thirty and forty,* the examination should be done within three months of the starting date and should include a resting electrocardiogram. Those between the *ages of forty-one and fifty-nine years* should also have an exercise electrocardiogram, using either the step, bicycle or treadmill technique. For the apparently healthy person *over age fifty-nine,* the physical examination needs to be done within two weeks of starting the fitness program and should include a resting and an exercise electrocardiogram. The person with known *coronary heart disease* should be at least two months postinfarction before starting a long-range conditioning program involving other than walking. If such a program is limited to walking, it can be performed without medical supervision, provided a screening examination does not detect heart failure or serious cardiac rhythm disturbances. The patient should be taught to check his own radial or carotid pulse rate and should limit the intensity of walking to that producing a pulse rate of less than 120 beats per minute. He should be instructed to wait two hours after a meal before walking, to avoid walking in extremes of weather, and to stop promptly if he experiences any chest discomfort.

Postcoronary patients who wish to undergo more strenuous forms of conditioning, including jogging and swimming, should do so under the direct supervision of medical or highly-skilled paramedical personnel, and in the presence of emergency resuscitation equipment (including a defibrillator). We prefer a defibrillator which has "print-out paddles", and frequently spot check cardiac rates and rhythm by this method. The ten absolute contraindications to such forms of activity are as follows: [249,250]

1. Moderate to severe aortic outflow obstruction (supravalvular, valvular, subvalvular)
2. Congestive heart failure
3. Acute infectious disease, including active myocarditis
4. Rapidly progressive angina pectoris
5. Acute myocardial infarction
6. Dissecting aortic aneurysms
7. Thrombophlebitis
8. Poorly controlled supraventricular rhythm disorders (as rapid atrial fibrillation), serious ventricular rhythm disorders (as paroxysmal tachycardia, multifocal premature beats or uniform premature beats occurring in pairs or at a frequency of more than six/minute), and fixed-rate cardiac pacemakers
9. Severe systemic arterial hypertension (systolic pressure 200 mm Hg, diastolic pressure >110 mmHg)
10. Cyanotic congenital heart disease

There are a number of *relative contraindications* to exercise training in which the possible benefits of exercise must be carefully weighed against the risks involved. These relative contraindications include pulmonary hypertension, ventricular aneurysms, poorly-controlled metabolic diseases such as diabetes mellitus or thyroid disorders, and toxemias of pregnancy. In addition, *special consideration* should be given to patients with cardiac pacemakers, congenital heart disease other than the cyanotic variety, and any form of chronic disease that might make it difficult to achieve a training effect. Such diseases include chronic renal or hepatic disorders, arthritis and musculoskeletal problems, and neuropsychiatric disorders. The cardiac exercise class should not be permitted to become a "catch-all" for severe cardiac problems in which there is no other form of therapy. Patients with severe angina pectoris, three-vessel coronary disease on angiography, and an akinetic myocardium on ventriculography are not candidates for coronary bypass surgery and neither are they candidates for a progressive exercise rehabilitation program.

Upon entering the exercise program the patient must be advised to adhere to the exercise prescription. Unless this is done, patients have a tendency to keep up with advanced members of the group and to see how many repetitions of one exercise can be performed without serious sequelae. The group supervisors must be on the lookout for such instances and should report them immediately to the physician in charge. We make it a routine practice before each exercise session of asking each participant whether he (or she) has experienced chest pain within the past twenty-four hours. Several of our participants, after having been up most of the night before with prolonged chest pain, will report to the gym and try to "work the pain out." It requires patient education (and re-education), daily questioning and careful supervision to keep such instances from occurring. In our program, patients are not permitted to exercise if they have experienced any unusual type of recent chest pain. They are advised instead to promptly get in touch with their personal physician.

There are several basic rules that exercise participants are expected to adhere to. They are advised against exercising within two hours of a large meal and to refrain from coffee, tea, cigarettes and alcohol during the same time segment. They should warm-up for five minutes before the inception of exercise and should cool-down for the same period of time after exercise before showering. The latter should be done using lukewarm water. The "buddy" system is used in the dressing room so that no individual is alone in the shower or dressing room. The doors on the toilets should not be locked from the inside, for in one program a patient suffered a cardiac arrest while straining during defecation.

The rules are applied in an inconspicuous manner. One does not wish for the participants to look upon the exercise class as an extention of the coronary care unit, but rather as a place to enjoy meaningful and pleasurable activity and social exchange. There are several ways to enhance the program and thereby to improve the patient adherence. One is for the physician and paramedical team members to actually participate with the class. This not only makes it easier to know each member, but it emphasizes that the medical staff practices what it preaches. It is important for the medical staff to know the names of all class members and for the members to learn the names of each other. Periodic group photographs, with an accompanying name list, help in this direction. New members should be introduced to at least several of the veterans so that they feel more comfortable in the initial phases of the program, the period in which the drop-out rate tends to be the highest. The patient's spouse is encouraged to also participate in the program, (Fig. 15) provided that she obtains permission from her personal physician. In some instances children are likewise permitted to exercise with their parents. This enhances adherence, emphasizes the use of exercise as a preventive health measure, and can lead to stronger family ties. By including coronary-prone members in the same class with the postcoronary patients, one can impress upon the former the importance of preventive cardiology. When asked in the locker room when he

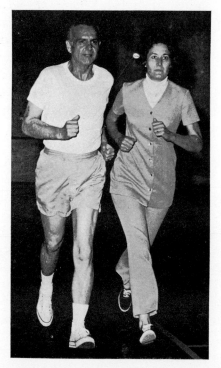

Figure 15. A postmyocardial infarction patient and his wife jog together in the gymnasium exercise program.

had his "event," one coronary-prone member promptly replied that he had not had one "yet." After collecting his thoughts, he indicated that hopefully his participation in the rehabilitation program might considerably decrease his chances of ever having one.

*Chapter VII*

# CORONARY RISK FACTOR DETECTION AND EXERCISE PRESCRIPTION IN A PREVENTIVE CARDIOLOGY CLINIC

A LTHOUGH AN ASSOCIATION for the "prevention and relief" of heart disease was started in 1920,[250] the practice of preventive cardiology has long been neglected, prompting Dr. Irvine Page to make the following statement: "Someday we may even realize that it is vastly more important, if not glamorous, to prevent atherosclerosis rather than repair the damage after it is done." [251] In an attempt to fulfill a need in this area, the Preventive Cardiology Clinic was formed in July, 1972. It is a highly specialized center with a staff that includes an attending cardiologist, an exercise physiologist, a consultant orthopedist (with a practice limited to sports medicine), dieticians and nursing personnel. A local and national committee of physicians and physiologists assist the clinic in providing the broad professional competency necessary to meet the objectives of preventive cardiology. The latter includes: (1) detection of early signs of coronary heart disease, (2) identification and modification of known risk factors that predispose a person to this disease, and (3) determination of an individual's physical work capacity (ie. the physiological evaluation of the oxygen transport system).

Each complete evaluation includes:

1. A comprehensive medical, physical activity and dietary history, using the problem-oriented method of medical record keeping.
2. A biochemical profile, including serum lipoprotein electrophoresis.
3. Body composition analysis (determination of lean body mass and percent body fat), using the skinfold caliper technique and sampling at ten sites.
4. Pulmonary function testing.
5. Personality-behavior pattern testing, using a modified Rosenman-Friedman questionnaire and structured interview.
6. A resting electrocardiogram.

84

7. A submaximal or maximal exercise stress test with continuous electrocardiographic monitoring and maximal oxygen uptake determination.

## Methods of Quantitating Coronary Risk

Several methods of quantitating coronary risk can be utilized. A simple method entails the completion of a risk factor questionnaire at the initial clinic visit (Table XIV). The points for various positive factors are totaled and the patient is placed in one of five categories (Table XV). While this provides a rough index of risk, there are certain obvious limitations. The main limitation is the lack of statistical support for the relative significance of each factor. For instance, it is arbitrary to say that the relative risk of a serum cholesterol level of 350 mg percent is the same as a cigarette intake in excess of two packs per day.

A more specific clinical index of coronary artery disease is that

TABLE XIV
CORONARY RISK FACTOR QUESTIONNAIRE

| *RISK FACTOR* | *POINTS* |
|---|---|
| 1. Cigarette Smoking | |
| (a) 2 packs/day | 7 |
| (b) 1–2 packs/day | 6 |
| (c) ½–1 pack/day | 5 |
| 2. Hypertension (systolic bp >150 or diastolic bp >90) | 5 |
| 3. Elevated serum cholesterol | |
| (a) 350 | 7 |
| (b) 300–350 | 6 |
| (c) 250–300 | 5 |
| (d) 225–250 | 3 |
| 4. Family history of coronary disease before age 55 | 4 |
| 5. Overweight >15% | 3 |
| 6. Elevated serum triglyceride | |
| (a) 300 | 5 |
| (b) 150–300 | 3 |
| 7. Diabetes mellitus | 3 |
| 8. Type A personality | 2 |
| 9. Abnormal EKG | 2 |
| 10. Enlarged heart on chest X-ray | 2 |
| 11. Low aerobic capacity | 3 |
| (no regular (3x week) endurance as swimming, jogging or bicycling) | |
| 12. Abnormal exercise stress test | 17 |

TABLE XV

CORONARY RISK CATEGORIES

| | |
|---|---|
| I. Very Low | (<6 points) |
| II. Low | (6–10 points) |
| III. Average | (11–15 points) |
| IV. Above average | (16–20 points) |
| V. Very high | (>20 points) |

used by Cohn *et al.*[251,253] at the Peter Bent Brigham Hospital. These investigators obtained multiple clinical parameters on a series of one hundred persons who were suspected of having underlying coronary heart disease. Coronary arteriograms were normal in 38 percent and abnormal (i.e. greater than 75 percent occlusion of one major artery) in 62 percent. Chemical parameters of statistical significance between the two groups included age, sex, history of ischemic episodes, resting electrocardiograms (pathologic Q-waves and ST-T abnormalities), postexercise electrocardiograms, serum lipoprotein and glucose levels, and graphic recordings (third and fourth heart sound recordings, apexcardiogram, left ventricular ejection time). Multiple discriminant analysis was used and each factor was given a numerical coefficient. The product of the latter times the coded value of each risk factor produced a numerical clinical index. Of sixty-two patients with coronary artery disease documented on arteriography, sixty-nine (97 percent) had clinical index values above one hundred points. Of the thirty-eight patients with normal coronary arteriograms, thirty-four (89 percent) had clinical indices below one hundred points. There were no false negatives in those patients whose clinical index was less than eighty points; that is, there were no significant abnormalities on coronary angiography in these patients. On the other hand, false positive results were seen in only 10 percent of those with indices ranging from one hundred to 120 points and less than 5 percent in those with indices above 120 points.

The practicality and simplicity of the clinical index point system can be seen in the following example:

A fifty-year-old executive with vague chest pain unrelated to exertion was evaluated at the clinic. His resting electrocardiogram revealed ST-T abnormalities. The maximal treadmill stress test showed down-

sloping S-T segment depression of 1.0 mm. The lipoprotein electrophoresis indicated a type IV pattern. A two-hour postprandial blood
sugar was normal. A fourth heart sound was noted clinically and recorded during phonocardiography. His clinical index was calculated
as seen in Table XVI.

TABLE XVI

CLINICAL INDEX FOR CORONARY DISEASE DETECTION

| Variable | Coded value of variable | Numerical Coefficient | Points |
|---|---|---|---|
| 1. age | years | 0.7 | 0.7 x 50 = 35 |
| 2. sex | 0 = Female | 24 | 1 x 24 = 24 |
| | 1 = Male | | |
| 3. history of ischemia | 0 = atypical angina | 16 | 16 x 0 = 0 |
| | 1 = typical angina | | |
| | 3 = documented myocardial infarction | | |
| 4. resting ECG | 0 = normal | 2 | 2 x 1 = 2 |
| | 1 = ST-T abnormalities | | |
| | 3 = pathologic Q waves | | |
| 5. stress test ECG | 0 = negative | 14 | 14 x 2 = 28 |
| | 2 = positive | | |
| 6. lipoprotein and glucose | 0 = normal | 16 | 16 x 1 = 16 |
| | 1 = type II or IV lipoprotein and blood glucose abnormalities | | |
| 7. graphic recordings (apex- and phonocardiography and external carotid pulse tracings) | 0 = normal | 8 | 8 x 1 = 8 |
| | 1 = S4 and/or S3 sounds; abnormal "a" wave on apex; decreased left ventricular ejection time | | |
| | 3 = combinations of above | | |
| | Total | | 113 points |

This patient's point total would make him likely to have significant (greater than 75 percent) obstruction of at least one
major coronary vessel.

The original study of Cohen *et al.*[251] was done in retrospective
fashion. A prospective series, also on one hundred patients, revealed similar results. Thirty-one of thirty-four persons (91 percent) with clinical indices below one hundred points had normal
coronary arteriograms. Sixty-one of sixty-six patients (92 percent)
with clinical indices above one hundred points had significant

abnormalities on coronary angiography, including forty-nine (74 percent) with multivessel disease.

A more complex method of assessing future coronary risk is that of Keys *et al.*[252] which involves the use of a programing calculator. The probability of developing future coronary disease was estimated by the multiple logistic equation using characteristics of age, serum cholesterol, cigarette smoking habits, body mass index and systolic blood pressure. Of 11,132 men, ages forty to fifty-nine years, who were followed for five years, 615 developed heart disease. There was high correlation between the number of predicted cases and the number of observed cases. Since the actual number of cases among American men was underpredicted, risk factors which were not measured or possibly not yet identified are implied.

A new booklet on risk factor quantitation has recently been published by the American Heart Association. Based on the Framingham data, it is easy to use and should be of assistance to the practicing physician.

### The Exercise Prescription

Since many of the clinic patients are young executives, airline pilots and various professional people, a major interest and emphasis of the center is exercise testing, and prescribing an exercise program that is specifically tailored to an individual's needs and desires.

At the consultation session, the cardiologist and physiologist review the accumulated data on coronary risk and fitness classification with the patient. The latter is taught that he has a maximum pulse rate based on age and degree of present physical conditioning, that this rate can be predicted from a chart, and that it can be more precisely measured by exercise stress-testing. He is further advised that to achieve a training effect he must perform endurance-type of activities that will maintain the pulse rate above 70 percent of the maximum rate for a total of one hundred to 140 minutes per week. If the person has not participated in any regular exercise program recently he is advised to build up to the one hundred to 140 minutes gradually and is given a schedule to guide him (Table XVII).

The exercise prescription is based upon the MET unit system,

TABLE XVII

CARDIOPULMONARY ENDURANCE EXERCISE SCHEDULE
FOR THE UNTRAINED PERSON

| | | |
|---|---|---|
| Week 1–2 | 20 minutes (at the prescribed MET unit level) | 3 times/week |
| Week 3–4 | 20 minutes | 4 times/week |
| Week 5–6 | 25 minutes | 4 times/week |
| Week 7–8 | 25 to 35 minutes | 4 times/week |
| Week 9 and beyond | Select one of the following: | |
| | (1) 20 minutes, 7 days/week | |
| | (2) 23 minutes, 6 days/week | |
| | (3) 28 minutes, 5 days/week | |
| | (4) 35 minutes, 4 days/week | |
| | (5) 45 minutes, 3 days/week | |

one MET unit being the amount of energy expended at rest multiplied by a factor of 1.1. If a person's maximum tolerance for work, as measured on the treadmill, is 10 MET units, the exercise prescription is for 70 percent of this value, (or 7 MET units). In order to make the endurance exercise more enjoyable, this patient may choose from a list of activities which are comparable to a given number of MET units (Table XVIII). Obviously, if someone strongly dislikes jogging, he is unlikely to adhere to a regimen in which this form of activity is emphasized.

Patients are instructed in the self-determination of pre- and postexercise pulse rates. They are asked to record this on a postcard, along with the frequency of exercise per week, and mail it to the clinic. Repeat treadmill testing is done three months after initial evaluation and at least annually thereafter. The maximal oxygen uptake value is recorded on a graph (Fig. 16) in order to better enable a patient to follow his progress and to see how his fitness level compares to others in the same group.

For a baseline maintenance exercise regimen, exercises that can be done alone are stressed. These include brisk walking, jogging, swimming, cycling, rope-skipping and bench stepping. Except for swimming, none of these activities require a special facility. A certain amount of skill is required only for swimming, unless one has never ridden a bicycle nor skipped rope as a youth. These activities should constitute the majority of time spent in cardiopulmonary conditioning. As previously mentioned, they should be supplemented by some of the group activities in the

TABLE XVIII
## CLASSIFICATION OF ACTIVITY BY MET UNITS [198]

| *3–4 METS* | *6–7 METS* (continued) |
|---|---|
| Walking (3 MPH) | Tennis (singles) |
| Cycling (6 MPH) | Badminton (competition) |
| Softball (excluding pitcher) | Swimming (1.6 MPH) |
| Dancing (moderate) | Step-up (24 steps/minute, 32 cm height) |
| Pitching horse shoes | 7 METS |
| Golf (pulling cart) | Double Master's test |
| Volleyball (6-man, not vigorous) | |
| Badminton (doubles) | |
| Steps (24 steps/minute, 12 cm height) | *7–8 METS* |
| 4 METS | Jogging (5 MPH) |
| Treadmill (2 MPH, 3.5% grade) | Cycling (12 MPH) |
| 3 METS | Swimming (side stroke, 1 MPH) |
| | Treadmill (3 MPH, 10% grade) |
| *4–5 METS* | 7 METS |
| Tennis (doubles) | Basketball (moderate) |
| Walking (3½ MPH) | Touch football |
| Cycling (8 MPH) | Skiing (hard, downhill) |
| Ping Pong | Horseback riding (gallop) |
| Golf (carrying clubs) | Mountain hiking (without back pack) |
| Raking leaves | Step-up (24 steps/minute, 35 cm height) |
| Calisthenics (in general) | 8 METS |
| Rowing (noncompetitive) | |
| Dancing (vigorous) | *8–9 METS* |
| Step-up (24 steps/minute, 18 cm height) | Jogging (5½ MPH) |
| 5 METS | Cycling (13 MPH) |
| Treadmill (2 MPH, 7% grade) 4 METS | Fencing |
| | Basketball (vigorous) |
| *5–6 METS* | Handball |
| Walking (4 MPH) | Paddleball |
| Cycling (10 MPH) | Step-up (30 steps/minute, 28 cm height) |
| Ice Skating | 9 METS |
| Roller skating | *10–11 METS* |
| Horseback riding (trot) | Running (6 MPH) 10 METS |
| Swim (1 MPH) | Handball (vigorous) |
| Step-up (24 steps/minute, 25 cm height) | Paddleball (vigorous) |
| 6 METS | Swimming (back stroke, 1.6 MPH) |
| Treadmill (2 MPH, 10.5% grade) | Step-up (30 steps/minute, 36 cm height) |
| 5 METS | 11 METS |
| | Treadmill (3.4 MPH, 14% grade) |
| *6–7 METS* | 10 METS |
| Walking (5 MPH) | |
| Cycling (11 MPH) | *12+ METS* |
| Water skiing | Running (8 MPH) 13½ METS |
| Lawn-mowing (hand mower) | Rowing (11 MPH) 13½ METS |
| Skiing (towing or easy downhill) | Step-up (30 steps/minute, 40 cm height) |
| Square dancing | 12 METS |
| | Treadmill (3.4 MPH, 18% grade) |
| | 12 METS |

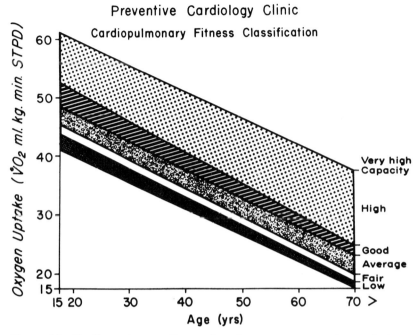

Figure 16. Cardiorespiratory fitness, based on oxygen uptake analysis, as plotted on an age-adjusted graph.

cases where that is possible. For example, the businessman who travels extensively could easily pack a jump-rope or a pair of walking or jogging shoes. He might swim at a motel pool or perhaps carry a stationary cycle in the trunk of his car. Easier still, he could measure the elevation of a certain object, such as a chair or stool in his room, and use it for bench-stepping exercise. A minimum of time is required, but this is well worth the investment.

The following four case histories best exemplify the nature of the preventive cardiology evaluation and the method of exercise prescription:

### Case 1

A forty-five-year-old airline pilot was evaluated for coronary risk and level of physical fitness. The history revealed sporadic jogging in the past and a fatal myocardial infarction in a brother, age fifty-three years. The physical examination indicated mild hypertension and excess body weight. The biochemical profile indicated an elevated fasting blood sugar (144 mg %), serum cholesterol (321 mg %) and serum triglyceride (369 mg %). The resting electrocardiogram was normal. The patient underwent treadmill testing by the Bruce method, reaching a maximum heart rate of 170 beats per minute before onset of fatigue. The S-T segment was depressed 1.0 mm in a horizontal fashion during the latter stages of exercise but was upsloping in the post-exercise tracings. The maximum oxygen uptake was 35 ml/kg/min., placing him in an average category for his age group. The personality pattern questionnaire was suggestive of a Type B pattern. Body composition analysis by the skin fold technique indicated that fat constituted 19 percent of his total body weight. A three-day dietary diary was assessed and indicated a daily caloric consumption ranging between 4,000 to 5,000 calories.

A lipoprotein electrophoresis was subsequently obtained and was normal. A two-hour postprandial blood glucose was mildly elevated. Because of the positive exercise test, the patient was placed in the medically-supervised exercise class at Georgia Baptist Hospital. His nutritional prescription called for a 1,400-calorie, fat-controlled diet which he and his wife were instructed in. When retested three months later, the amount of body fat decreased from 19 percent to 16 percent (of total weight). The oxygen uptake was 43.19 ml/kg/min. (vs. 35.9 ml/kg/min. initially). The serum triglyceride showed a 50 percent decrease, while the cholesterol diminished by 25 percent; more significantly, the exercise electrocardiogram showed no evidence of ischemia.

## Case 2

A forty-year-old writer was seen for a routine screening evaluation. His father had experienced a myocardial infarction at age sixty-two years, as did a half-brother at age forty-seven years. The resting blood pressure was mildly elevated (145/100 mm Hg.) The serum cholesterol was 283 mg % and the triglyceride was 143 mg %. The resting electrocardiogram was normal. The patient completed eight minutes of the Bruce treadmill test, reaching a maximum heart rate of 180 beats per minute. There were junctional S-T segment changes on the electrocardiogram during exercise but no evidence of ischemia. The maximum oxygen consumption of 25 ml/kg/min. was very low. Twenty-one percent of his total body weight was fat, indicating the need to lose twenty pounds of body fat. He was advised of having five coronary risk factors (excess fat, very low aerobic capacity, elevated serum cholesterol, systemic arterial hypertension and a family history of coronary disease).

He was placed on a fat and calorie-restricted diet and a home jogging program, working up to one-and-one-half miles per day over a six-week period. A friend was instructed in blood pressure recording and a diary was kept. When retested three months later he had lost fourteen pounds of fat weight and his oxygen consumption had increased to 31 ml/kg/min., a 16 percent increment. The blood pressure diary showed an average home reading of 130/85 mm Hg. The serum cholesterol had decreased to 258 mg %, a 25 mg % fall.

## Case 3

A fifty-seven-year-old company president underwent coronary risk assessment and exercise testing. He had been an Olympic-caliber athlete as a youth and had smoked cigarettes for thirty pack-years, quitting in 1957. Both parents lived beyond their eightieth year. He currently exercised an average of three times per week on a treadmill and on weight-training machines. He had been given clofibrate for hypercholesterolemia two years previously.

The physical examination was normal except for a midsystolic ejection click at the cardiac apex. The serum cholesterol was moderately elevated at 276 mg %. The resting electrocardiogram was normal as was a chest x-ray. He progressed to the fourth stage of the Bruce treadmill test with a maximum heart rate of 175 beats per minute. The exercise electrocardiogram was normal and the maximum oxygen consumption was 43 ml/kg/min., a very high level for his age group. Since his maximum MET unit of exercise tolerance was 12.3, he was advised to exercise at a level of 9 MET units in hopes of maintaining his excellent level of conditioning. The clofibrate dosage was increased and nutritional counseling was obtained with the objective of reducing the serum cholesterol level to less than 220 mg %. He was advised to undergo exercise stress testing on an annual basis.

## Case 4

A fifty-one-year-old businessman was evaluated because of rather vague anterior chest pain. The history was significant in that his father died at age sixty-one years of a myocardial infarction. The physical examination was unremarkable except for excess body weight and a resting blood pressure of 190/120 mm Hg. On skin fold assessment, the percentage of total weight as fat was 22.5 percent. The cholesterol was moderately elevated (338 mg %) and the triglyceride was significantly elevated (486 mg %). The resting electrocardiogram was normal. The patient completed seven minutes of the Bruce test, attaining a peak pulse rate of 135 per minute and a blood pressure of 190/112 mm Hg. The S-T segment was depressed 2 mm during and immediately postexercise (Fig. 17), indicative of ischemia. The maximal oxygen

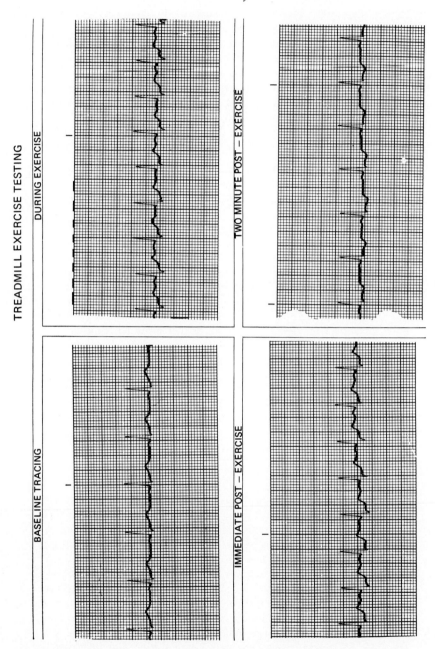

Figure 17. A positive exercise stress test on a fifty-one-year-old businessman.

consumption was extremely low at 13.9 ml/kg/min. The patient was advised of the multiple coronary risk factors. In view of the positive exercise electrocardiogram, he was entered in the medically-supervised exercise program and started on both antihypertensive and lipid-lowering agents. Six weeks later, while on a golfing vacation, he experienced several bouts of exercise-induced chest pain. An electrocardiogram, taken the following day, revealed inferior wall injury which subsequently evolved into an extensive anterior and inferior infarction. His two-week hospital course was uneventful and upon discharge he was begun on the home walking regimen. Two months later he underwent an evaluation before re-entering the outpatient gymnasium program. His body fat had decreased 3 percent. The serum cholesterol had fallen from 388 mg % to 335 mg %; the triglyceride level was now 220 mg %. The exercise electrocardiogram continued to show significant S T segment depression. He began at a low level of gymnasium exercise and has progressed to brisk walking and slow jogging activities with no adverse signs or symptoms.

# Chapter VIII

# POSTINFARCTION REHABILITATION:

# HOSPITAL PHASE

UNTIL THE LAST decade, the general consensus among physicians treating patients with coronary heart disease was that physical activity had deleterious effects in the clinical setting of recent myocardial infarction. The treatment was rather stereotyped in that most acute coronary victims could expect up to six to eight weeks of bed rest within the hospital and at home postdischarge. This period of strict bed rest was based upon early studies of Levine and Brown [255] dealing with the duration of the healing process. In 1929 these authors stated that activity too soon postinfarction could lead to mural thrombus formation, aneurysm development or myocardial rupture. As the maximum healing process, including the formation of scar tissue, took place within six to eight weeks postinfarction, it seemed reasonable to markedly reduce myocardial oxygen demands and cardiac work during this time segment.

With the advent of cardiac catheterization and other refined techniques in hemodynamic assessment it became obvious that there were certain disadvantages of maintaining a cardiac patient in a recumbent position for prolonged periods of time. Coe [256] found that cardiac work increased 29 percent when normal subjects or cardiac patients were moved from sitting to recumbent positions. The latter position resulted in an augmentation of venous return, increasing contractility through the Frank-Starling mechanism. The failing heart, or the heart with a compromised coronary circulation, could be unduly stressed by prolonged recumbency.

There has been recent controversy, particularly in the British medical literature, as to not only the optimal length of hospitalization postinfarction but also the veracity of hospitalization itself. A randomized study [257] was set up to compare home care by the family doctor and hospital treatment. The latter involved an initial period of observation in a coronary care unit. Participating in the study were 458 English general practitioners who allocated 343 cases at random to the two treatment groups. The groups did not differ significantly with respect to age, prior diagnosis of angina pectoris, previous myocardial infarction or history of hypertension. The groups were also similar with respect to the prevalence of hypotension when initially examined. Of 169 hospitalized patients, the twenty-eight day mortality rate was 14.2 percent compared to 9.8 percent for the 174 patients who were treated at home. Although the results certainly provide food for thought in an era of super mechanization and medical gadgetry, the study had certain definite drawbacks which bear mentioning. For instance, a number of patients initially treated at home were later transferred to the hospital, clouding the issue considerably since they were still considered to be in the home care group. Moreover, the location and severity of the infarctions were not compared in the two groups, nor was analysis made of the time lapse between the onset of symptoms and the initial call for medical help.

When looking at studies such as this, one needs to be highly critical. It is likewise important for the practitioner to draw upon his past experience and to employ a little common sense. It is certainly not difficult for most practicing physicians to recall numerous instances of life-threatening cardiac arrhythmias which were promptly recognized and treated in the coronary care unit and which probably would have resulted in the patient's demise had they occurred at home.

A more reasonable controversy centers around the question of early versus late mobilization and discharge postmyocardial infarction. Wenger *et al.*[258] published the results of a questionnaire as to the current physician practice in managing uncomplicated myocardial infarction patients. The questionnaire was sent to 1200 general practitioners, 1200 internists and 1200 cardiologists. The 69 percent who responded managed 70,000 patients with acute myocardial infarctions during 1970. The responses were similar for the three groups in the 95 percent of the patients were hospitalized for twenty-one days; most were permitted to sit in a chair on the eighth hospital day and to walk in the room on the fourteenth day. Dr. Geoffrey Rose [259] recently made the following statement pertaining to old traditions and modern doubts of in-hospital care:

> Physicians have always been very cautious in their management of patients with myocardial infarction. We are less upset if our patient dies in bed than if he dies while walking in the ward or street, for in confining him to bed we feel that at least we did everything possible.

But have we? In 1952, Levine and Lown [260] published the results of arm chair rather than bed rest treatment for seventy-three patients with myocardial infarction, indicating that there were no evident ill effects from such therapy. They also pointed out the various hazards of immobilization, including rapid muscle wasting, decreased pulmonary ventilation, impaired exercise tolerance and loss of normal postural vasomotor reflexes. The latter was clearly demonstrated by Fareeduddin and Abelmann.[261] They reported that five of ten patients treated for nine to twenty-four days with strict bed rest had transient systemic blood pressure decreases of more than 38 mm Hg during fifteen minutes of passive upright tilt to seventy degrees. This response was abolished after a period of full ambulation and was not observed in eight patients who were treated with modified bed rest. Such a significant fall in blood pressure could be catastrophic to a patient with a compromised myocardial blood supply in that it could lead to reinfarction or to extention of the initial infarction.

Saltin *et al.*[24] have carried out extensive studies on the effect of a twenty-day period of bed rest on five normal subjects ages nineteen to twenty-one. Two of the subjects were very active physically prior to the study, while the remainder had been essentially sedentary. The maximum oxygen uptake fell from a mean of 3.3 liters/minute before bed rest to 2.43 liters/minute. During supine exercise on a bicycle ergometer at 600 kpm/minute, the stroke volume decreased 25 percent and the heart rate increased from an average of 129 beats/minute to 154 beats/minute. An oxygen uptake that could normally be attained at a heart rate of

145 beats/minute now required a rate of 180 beats/minute after bed rest. During maximal treadmill testing the cardiac output fell 26 percent after bed rest (from 20 to 14.8 liters/minute). This was attributed to a reduction in stroke volume since the maximal arteriovenous oxygen difference and the maximal heart rate was not altered.

Numerous recent reports have dealt with the results of early mobilization and discharge after myocardial infarction. In Northern Ireland, Adgey [262] reported 102 patients who were hospitalized for an average period of thirteen days postinfarction. Over a two-week period after discharge there was no mortality and no apparent morbidity that might have been prevented by a more prolonged hospital stay. Takkunen *et al.*[263] in Finland, compared 146 patients who were mobilized after three to seven days in the hospital and discharged between twelve to sixteen days with 108 patients who were bed-ridden for seven to fourteen days and hospitalized for twenty-one to twenty-eight days. There was no significant difference when the mortality rates were assessed at seven days and again at thirty days postdischarge. This study had the limitations of not being randomized and not including long-term results. Tucker *et al.*[264] (England) were more aggressive and discharged 89 percent of 289 postinfarction patients by the tenth hospital day. Of this group, 7.6 percent were readmitted during a six-week follow-up period and 6.7 percent of the discharged patients died. The authors seemed encouraged by this approach and noted that 62 percent of the patients were back at work five months after their infarction. The results and conclusions are, however, a little bothersome for several reasons. First, 38 percent of their patients were still out of work five months postinfarction, a figure which exceeds that in many institutions. Second, in the absence of a randomized control group, the possibility exists that the six-week postdischarge mortality and morbidity rates might exceed that of a group hospitalized for a longer period of time.

Fortunately there are two recent reports of fairly well-controlled studies which may serve as guidelines. Harpur *et al.*[265] studied 199 patients with uncomplicated myocardial infarctions. All were given seven days of bed rest and then allocated into either Plan A or Plan B. In the former, patients were mobilized on day eight and discharged on the fifteenth hospital day. In Group B, patients were mobilized on day twenty-one and discharged on the twenty-eighth hospital day. All patients were encouraged to return to work one month after discharge. The groups were well-matched with respect to previous cardiovascular history, age, sex, interval from onset of pain to admission, and site of infarction. In the first eight months after infarction, the early and late mobilization groups did not differ significantly with respect to cardiac mortality or morbidity, congestive heart failure, serious arrhythmias or the development of ventricular aneurysm formation. There was a significant difference in the "return to work" rate two months after admission. In the early mobilization group 41 percent were back at work in two months versus only 17 percent of the late mobilization group. As Rose has pointed out, this study was not entirely free of selection bias in that patients were included in the early mobilization group only if they had been free of hypotension, congestive heart failure or serious arrhythmias in the preceeding five days.

Hutter *et al.*,[266] at the Massachusetts General Hospital, described a prospective randomized controlled study comparing a two-week and a three-week hospital stay in 138 patients with uncomplicated myocardial infarctions. The groups were comparable for age, sex, prior cardiovascular problems and location of infarction. During a six-month follow-up period there were no group differences in terms of coronary mortality or morbidity, aneurysm formation, psychological signs and symptoms, congestive heart failure and number returning to work. The authors concluded that there appeared to be no additional benefit from a three-week hospital course as compared to a two-week period for patients with uncomplicated myocardial infarctions.

Rose [259] has summarized the controversies of early versus late mobilization and has offered the following suggested policy:

1. Until further controlled studies are available, the coronary patient free of severe pain or shock may be treated with bed or chair rest for the first seven days of hospitalization. The legs should be exercised daily and a bedside commode is preferred over a bedpan.
2. Beginning on the eighth hospital day the "good risk" patient (devoid of persistent pain, congestive heart failure and ventricular

arrhythmias) can be allowed to ambulate in the ward. He can be discharged several days later and can soon return to work.

3. Patients who do not fall in the "good risk" group must be managed on a highly individualized basis. Since this is such a diverse group, fixed rules do not apply.

At Georgia Baptist Hospital, the cardiac rehabilitation team sees only those patients whose physicians fill out the referral sheet (Table XIX). The team consists of a physician and nurse coordinators working in conjunction with the physical therapist, dietician, chaplain, social worker and pharmacologist (Fig. 18).

TABLE XIX
CARDIAC REHABILITATION REFERRAL SHEET

DOCTOR:_____  DATE:_____

PATIENT:_____  ROOM:_____  AGE:_____

PLEASE CHECK:

_____I would like to refer this patient to the cardiac rehabilitation program.

_____I would *not* like to refer this patient to the cardiac rehabilitation program.

*REHABILITATION SERVICES DESIRED*

I. INDIVIDUAL PATIENT AND FAMILY CONFERENCES (to begin now and progress after the acute phase)

_____Dietary history, analysis and instruction

_____Risk factors (smoking, diet, exercise, weight, blood lipids)

_____Instruction concerning current cardiac problems

_____Religious counseling (via hospital chaplain)

_____Psychological testing (Minnesota Multiphasic Personality Inventory or Behavior Type Screening Survey)

II. PHYSICAL ACTIVITY PROGRAM (directed by the cardiac rehabilitation physician)

_____Physical therapy

_____Progressive daily activity [ie: self grooming→chair→walking (a list of these progressive activities is posted on each ward) ]

_____Telemetry exercise monitoring _____ with stairs

_____Discuss the outpatient exercise program

_____(a) First 3 months after discharge

III. PATIENT AND FAMILY GROUP CONFERENCES (to begin in post coronary phase)

_____Diet instruction    _____Coronary heart disease

_____Risk factors    _____Vocational rehabilitation counseling

IV. FOLLOW-UP

_____Home visit

_____Return to hospital for group conferences

_____Health agency referral

SIGNED: _____

TABLE XX

CARDIAC REHABILITATION INPATIENT EXERCISE REGIMEN*
GEORGIA BAPTIST HOSPITAL—ATLANTA MEDICAL CENTER

| Step | Where & When | Exercise | Activity |
|---|---|---|---|
| 1 | CCU (monitor) | Passive ROM to all extremities (5 x each) in bed. Active planter and dorsiflexion of ankles. (10 x each t.i.d.) | OOB to chair, 15 min. B.I.D. or commode Feed self. |
| 2 | CCU (monitor) Day 3–4 | Partial assistance in flexion, extension and rotation of shoulders, elbows, hips, knees and ankles. (4 x each q.d.) | Wash hands and face, brush teeth. Sitting in chair 15 min. t.i.d. |
| 3 | Telemetry unit. Day 5–7 | Minimal resistance to active ROM (shoulders, elbows, hips, knees, ankles) (5 x each q.d.) | Change gown plus steps 1–2 |
| 4 | Ward Day 8–10 | Moderate resistance to active ROM. With hands on shoulder circle elbows (5 x each) | Steps 1–3 plus: dress, shave, comb hair (sitting) Walk back and forth in room (2 x q.i.d.) |
| 5 | Ward Day 11–12 | Above plus walk to bathroom and back under observation. (p.r.n.) | Step 1–4 plus: Stand at sink to shave. May bathe legs. |
| 6 | Ward Day 13–14 (telemetry during exercise only) | Standing (a) arm and shoulder 3x (b) lat. bend 2x (c) knee raise 2x Supine in bed (a) bent leg raise 2x (b) str. leg raise 2x Side (a) leg raise 2x | Bathe in tub or shower. Walk to waiting room and sit for 15 min. 1x/d (telemetry) |
| 7 | Ward Day 15–16 | Step 6 plus: sitting on flat bed touch toes 2x and twist trunk 2x qid | Walk to waiting room 2x/d. Sit up most of the day |
| 8 | Ward Day 17–18 | All of above—3 half knee bends while standing | Walk length of hall 1x/d. Walk down flight of stairs with therapist. Take elevator up. |
| 9 | Ward Day 19–20 | All of above b.i.d. | Walk length of hall (50 ft.) 2x/d. Walk down two flights of stairs and take elevator up. |
| 10 | Ward Day 21 | All of above b.i.d. | Walk length of hall (50 ft.) 3x/d. Walk down and up one flight of stairs. |

TABLE XX—Continued

| Step | Where & When | Exercise | Activity |
|------|--------------|----------|----------|

CCU = coronary care unit
OOB = out of bed
ROM = range of motion
t.i.d. = three times daily
b.i.d. = two times daily
q.d. = daily
p.r.n. = as needed
q.i.d. = four times daily
x = times
d = day

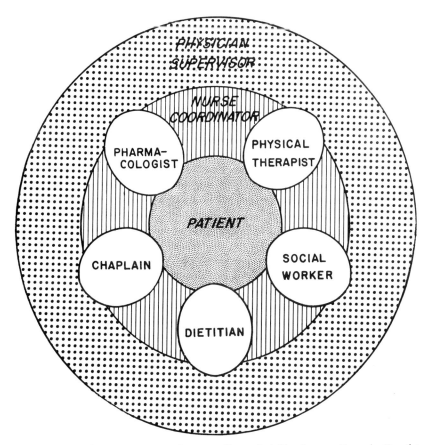

Figure 18. The team approach to cardiac rehabilitation at Georgia Baptist Hospital.

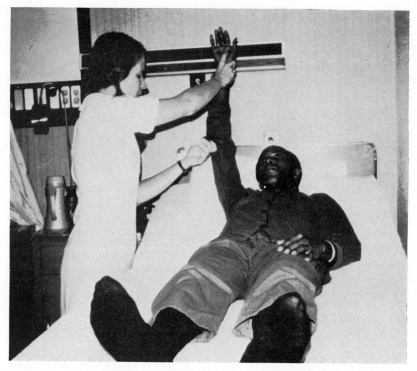

Figure 19. Passive bed exercise in the coronary care unit, supervised by the
physical therapist.

The pharmacologist reviews the medication list on all patients,
looking for possible adverse interactions, and counsels the patients
as to drug mechanisms and potential side effects. The physical
therapist follows a modification of the Emory University inpatient
activity regimen (Table XX). It is similar to the suggestions of
Rose in that most patients can be sitting in a chair while still in
the coronary care unit. The patients begin to ambulate on the
seventh hospital day and prior to discharge at day fourteen to
sixteen are walking in the halls and climbing one or two flights
of stairs under telemetry monitoring. The patients perform first
passive and then active bed exercise under the supervision of the
physical therapist (Fig. 19). The activities are terminated if the
pulse rate is greater than 115 beats/minute or if ectopic beats
occur. At Grady Memorial Hospital the Emory regimen has been

used on over 2000 patients [267] with only one mishap, that being an instance of ventricular fibrillation during passive range of motion exercise that was promptly terminated by electrical defibrillation.

Patients are encouraged to flex and extend the feet and knees on an hourly basis. To do so on a once or twice-daily schedule is probably ineffective as suggested by the study of Browse,[268] who measured calf blood flow with venous-occlusion plethysmography. The blood flow increased significantly following leg exercises but returned to the resting basal level within one hour of rest. We also encourage the use of elastic stockings which have been known to increase the speed of venous return from ankle to groin as measured by the $I^{125}$—labeled hippuran injection technique.[269] Other investigators, however, have used the tagged fibrinogen scanning technique in postoperative patients, and have demonstrated counts in the lower legs indicative of venous thrombosis in 32 percent of both control and elastic stocking groups; [270] hence, more studies involving postcoronary patients are needed before the true value of this simple form of preventive therapy can be assessed. Multiple studies have shown that minidose subcutaneous heparin, given before surgery and continued for several doses after, is effective in preventing calf-vein thrombosis.[271] Handley [272] has shown that this regimen is not effective in patients with acute myocardial infarction, attributing this to the fact that the therapy in these instances is started after the event that initiated the thrombosis. Wray *et al.*[273] randomly allocated ninety-two consecutive patients with acute myocardial infarction into a control group and an anticoagulated group. The latter consisted of heparin for the initial forty-eight hours, followed by Coumadin®. Both groups underwent active physiotherapy from the onset of admission and were mobilized to a chair within seven days of the acute event. The groups were well-matched in the severity of cardiac illness as assessed by a coronary prognostic index. All patients were given intravenous injections of labeled fibrinogen and the lower extremities were scanned daily, looking for evidence of venous thrombosis. Daily chest x-rays were done on both groups and the last fifty patients in the study all had lung scans on the tenth hospital day. The group receiving the anticoagulants had a 6.5

percent incidence of calf vein thrombosis as compared to a 22 percent incidence in the control group. The thrombosis development occurred remarkably early in the hospital course as more than 60 percent developed within seventy-two hours of the clinical onset of infarction. This would suggest that the infarction itself, rather than a period of prolonged immobilization, was the precipitating factor. It is of interest that the thrombi were confined to calf veins in all instances of both control and treatment patients. Moreover, clinically important pulmonary emboli did not occur in either group. It is possible that the active physical therapy and early mobilization regimen played some role in limiting the extention of thrombosis formation. As a result of the study, the authors now reserve anticoagulant therapy for those postinfarction patients who exhibit clinical evidence of deep vein thrombosis and those patients who are confined to bed for more than one week.

At Georgia Baptist Hospital most patients are anticoagulated with warfarin at least during the hospital phase of a myocardial infarction. Elastic stockings are commonly utilized in addition to the frequent leg exercises which are performed in the bed. We occasionally place a football or a soccerball at the foot of the bed, (ala Dr. Henry Marriott) and encourage the patients to move the ball about frequently with their feet.

In addition to the inpatient physical program there are three other general groups of services which are available to the patient who is referred to the cardiac rehabilitation team. *Group I* consists of individual patient and family conferences, and includes discussion and instructions in diet, coronary risk factors and current cardiac problems. Religious counseling and psychological testing are done in selected instances. All phases of activities within this group are conducted in the individual patient's room. *Group II* deals with group conferences pertaining to the pathophysiology of coronary atherosclerosis, the psychosocial aspects of coronary disease, diet and coronary risk factors (Fig. 20). These conferences are held in the cardiac rehabilitation office and make use of various audiovisual aids. The conferences are scheduled so that a different discussion is scheduled each week of the month. The patient's spouse and family are strongly urged to attend these sessions.

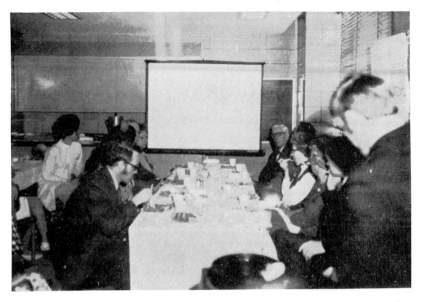

Figure 20. Family conference on the coronary risk factors held in the cardiac rehabilitation office.

*Group III* is the predischarge and follow-up phase. The former includes instructions on a home walking regimen (Table XXI) and general guidelines as to "do's" and "don'ts" during the early segment of home care. The topic of sexual activity is brought up by the rehabilitation team as patients are often embarrassed to initiate such discussion. The energy expenditure during this activity has been studied by Hellerstein and Friedman,[164] who found that the mean pulse rate during intercourse was 117 beats per minute in postinfarction patients. This is approximately the same energy cost of climbing two flights of stairs. Patients who have stable telemetry recordings during inhospital stair climbing are permitted to engage in sexual activities within a week after discharge. Group III activities also include the home visit which is made within the first twenty-four to forty-eight hours after discharge. The purpose of this visit is to directly assess the home situation and to consult on any problems that have arisen after discharge. A review of the patient's medications and dietary regimen is made, and a brief cardiopulmonary examination is

TABLE XXI

CARDIAC REHABILITATION HOME EXERCISE REGIMEN*

GEORGIA BAPTIST HOSPITAL—ATLANTA MEDICAL CENTER

| Week | Activity |
|------|----------|
| 1–3 | In-hospital exercise regimen |
| 4 | Walk 5 minutes at leisurely pace (1/4 mile) once per day |
| 5 | Walk 5 minutes at leisurely pace b.i.d. (1/2 mile) |
| 6 | Walk 10 minutes at leisurely pace (1/2 mile) once per day |
| 7 | Walk 10 minutes at leisurely pace (3/4 mile) once per day |
| 8 | Walk 15 minutes at leisurely pace (3/4 mile) once per day |
| 9 | Walk 15 minutes at leisurely pace (3/4 mile) once per day |
| 10 | Walk 20 minutes at leisurely pace (1 mile) once per day |
| 11 | Walk 20 minutes at moderate pace (1 1/3 mile) once per day |
| 12 | Walk 30 minutes at moderate pace (2 miles) once per day |
| 13 | Begin group activity program—Georgia Baptist Hospital |

*For 1st three months post-coronary incident          b.i.d. = two times daily

carried out. After the home visit a report is written for the rehabilitation files, and a copy is sent to the referring physician. If any problems are encountered which require immediate attention, the private physician is notified by telephone. The home visit provides a certain continuity to the inpatient rehabilitation program. When questions are answered and problems solved at an early point in the rehabilitation phase, the anxiety of the patient and family members is significantly decreased. All patients and family members are encouraged to call the cardiac rehabilitation department at any time they think the various team members might be of assistance.

To *summarize,* evidence is mounting that the uncomplicated postmyocardial infarction patient can be mobilized within the first few days of hospitalization and can be discharged after two weeks of hospital care. The latter is enhanced with a team approach to the various facets of the postinfarction state. In small community hospitals, an interested physician and nurse will suffice to guide the patient in secondary prevention measures and to assist him in handling the various psychosocial barriers that often accompany coronary disease. The hospital phase of a myocardial infarction can be a frightening experience, particularly to a person who has previously enjoyed good health. The fear of becoming a "cardiac invalid" is always present. The optimistic attitude of the rehabilitation team and the reassurrance of returning to an active, productive life has done much to allay the various apprehensions and anxieties of the coronary patient.

*Chapter IX*

# OUTPATIENT EXERCISE THERAPY FOR
# CORONARY DISEASE—A PRESCRIPTION

O VER THE PAST decade numerous investigators have expounded the benefits of increased activity and regular exercise for angina pectoris and the postmyocardial infarction state. The studies dealing with the largest number of patients are those of Hellerstein [75] and Gottheiner. [74] The latter reported a five-year follow-up on 1,103 male patients with coronary disease, 548 of whom had a previous myocardial infarction (although criteria for diagnosis were not listed). The exercise program began with several months of mild strength-building activities, which included weight lifting. Specifics of this initial program are not provided. After about nine months, the men engaged in rhythmic endurance exercises such as running, hiking, swimming, cycling, rowing and volleyball. Those who excelled in these activities and achieved a significant improvement in overall fitness then entered competitive team games. The participants in the general exercise program basically practiced on their own on a twice-daily schedule. There was obviously no medical supervision. Once a week, the men met as a group for instructions and practice. The most impressive results of the study are in the mortality rate data which was 3.6 percent for the entire group over the five-year period in contrast to 12 percent of a comparable nonexercised group of Israelis with previous myocardial infarctions. Gottheiner described other objective effects of training, such as reductions of resting heart rate and of resting and exercise blood pressure levels. In addition, there was less S-T segment depression on electrocardiograms taken during and immediately postexercise. Unfortunately, the complete data on these observations are not given, which makes the significance questionable. Hellerstein [75] noted the results of physical training on 656 middle-aged males, 203 of whom had angina pectoris and/or myocardial infarctions. An additional fifty-one men had resting or exercise stress test electrocardiograms compatible with silent coronary heart disease (utilizing the Minnesota code). Persons with valvular disease and uncompensated congestive failure were followed for an average of 2.7 years. They participated in at least a thrice-weekly exercise program and recreational activities. The latter included swimming, basketball, volleyball and use of a punching bag. Detailed results were presented on the first one hundred cardiac patients. The average weight loss was 2.5 kg. Sixty-five percent significantly improved their level of fitness, as measured by bicycle ergometric testing and oxygen consumption. Sixty-three percent showed improvement in their exercise electrocardiograms, mainly in terms of the initial slope and the junctional displacement of the S-T segment. The death rate for the exercise cardiac patients was 1.9 per one hundred patient years which was less than half the expected rate.

Rechnitzer *et al.*[76] reported the results of physical training in men with previous documented myocardial infarctions. There were two aspects to the study. One consisted of a comparison of the incidence of nonfatal recurrences and cardiac deaths between sixty-six men in the exercise group and seventy-one controls who were matched according to age, year of infarction and number of infarctions. All of the controls met the criteria for entry into the exercise program but did not for a variety of reasons (including job conflicts and personal physician disapproval). Over a seven year follow-up period the results were as follows:

|  | No | Nonfatal Recurrences | Cardiac Deaths |
|---|---|---|---|
| Exercise Group | 77 | 1 (1.3%) | 3 (3.9%) |
| Matched Control Group | 111 | 31 (28%) | 15 (11.8%) |

There were several weaknesses of the above study, however, which might have had a bearing on the results. For one thing, the control groups were not "true" controls in the sense that they were randomly assigned to the inactive group. It is possible that certain members of the control group had severe angina pectoris and did not enter the exercise program for this reason. Another vulnerable area of the study concerns the documentation of nonfatal recurrence of myocardial infarction. In some instances historical evidence supplied by the patient or his physician was utilized instead of much harder criteria such as enzyme and electrocardiographic changes. Still another deficit of the study was that the exercise and control groups were not matched for important risk factors such as cigarette smoking habits, hypertension, serum cholesterol levels and family history.

Kennedy *et al.*[274] reported the Mayo Clinic experience with eight men (ranging in age from forty-five to fifty-two years) who had stable angina pectoris. None of the men developed a myocardial infarction or died during the follow-up period. This has little significance, however, since the numbers are small, the follow-up was brief (one year) and a control group was not obtained. The study was of interest in that cardiac catheterization and coronary arteriography was performed prior to and at the completion of the one-year program. All patients had an increase in cardiac index after training (from a mean of 3.9 L/min/m² to 4.4 L/min/m²). Half of the patients showed a decrease in the magnitude of ischemic changes on follow-up exercise stress testing. Surprisingly, the left ventricular end-diastolic pressure increased in seven of the eight patients (from a mean of 16 mm Hg to 20 mm Hg). None of the individuals showed any increase in coronary collateral circulation posttraining, nor were such found in two other series.[154,275] Kattus *et al.*[276] noted enhanced collateral vessel development in three instances, however.

Perhaps the best-designed study of postinfarction physical training was that of Kentala [148] who randomly assigned patients into control or exercise groups. Of those who were discharged from the hospital, 158 men met the diagnostic criteria for a documented myocardial infarction. The exercise group was comprised of seventy-seven men while the control group numbered eighty-one men. The groups were similar regarding age, smoking habits, preinfarction physical activities, severity of infarction and serum cholesterol levels and lung vital capacities. Over a two-year follow-up period there were no group differences as to coronary mortality or morbidity. However, only ten of seventy-seven (13 percent) in the training group had attended at least 70 percent of the thrice-weekly exercise sessions by the end of one year, while eleven of eighty-one controls (14 percent) had engaged in a regular physical training program on their own. Therefore, it is not too surprising that group differences weren't detected. Those attending the exercise sessions on a regular basis showed significant weight loss, diminution of body fat and decrease in serum triglyceride levels. In addition, they demonstrated greater improvement in physical work capacity on exercise testing (p < .0025), had more success in giving up cigarette smoking, and had faster disappearances in Q-waves on the resting electrocardiogram.

A wide variety of exercise programs have been utilized by the various investigators. Unfortunately, none are clearly and concisely outlined in the literature. In view of this, the three types of outpatient exercise programs utilized at Georgia Baptist Hospital are presented in detail.

### Home Exercise Regimen (First Three Months Postcoronary Incident)

After completing the inpatient exercise and physical therapy program (Chapter VIII), most patients will be ready for a home walking program. The purpose of this is to very gradually increase their exercise tolerance for the more strenuous group activity program which begins three months postinfarction. The walking should be done on level ground and in good weather. Other guidelines (Chapter VI), should be followed as well. In inclement weather the patient may drive to an area shopping center and walk up and down the mall area. The specifics of the home regimen are seen in Table XXI.

### Home Exercise Regimen (Beginning Three Months Postcoronary Incident)

Certain patients are unable to participate in the physician-supervised exercise program beginning three months postinfarction, mainly because of logistical problems. For those who wish to advance to a higher level of endurance training, the program adapted from John L. Boyer, M.D. (San Diego, California) is recommended (Table XXII).[277] Before starting the program the individual is taught to check his own pulse rate. He is advised to not advance to the next stage (as from week one or two to week

TABLE XXII

CARDIAC REHABILITATION HOME EXERCISE PROGRAM
GEORGIA BAPTIST HOSPITAL—ATLANTA MEDICAL CENTER

| Week | Activity |
|---|---|
| 1–2 | Measure 1 mile distance with car. Walk to point and back (total of 2 miles) in 40 minutes. Pulse at end should be less than 115 per minute. |
| 3–4 | Measure 1.5 mile distance. Walk to point and back (3.0 miles) in 60 minutes. |
| 5–6 | Measure 2 miles distance. Walk to point and back (4.0 miles) in 72 minutes. |
| 7–9 | Measure 2 miles distance. Walk to point and back (4.0 miles) in 60 minutes. (15 minute mile pace) |
| 10–12 | Measure 2 miles distance. Walk to point and back (4.0 miles) in 56 minutes. (14 minute mile pace, just below a slow jog) |

TABLE XXIII

CORONARY GROUP WALK AND JOG CHART
PRIOR TO CALISTHENICS

| | (Perform minimum of 3 times per week) |
|---|---|
| Week 1 to 4 | Walk slowly 100 yards, walk briskly 100 yards, alternately for ¼ mile. |
| Week 5 to 8 | Walk slowly 100 yards, walk briskly 100 yards, alternately for ½ mile. |
| Week 9 to 12 | Walk slowly 100 yards, walk briskly 100 yards, jog 100 yards, alternately for ½ mile. |
| Week 13 to 15 | Walk briskly 200 yards, jog 200 yards, alternately for ¾ mile. |
| Week 16 to 24 | Jog 400 yards, walk 200 yards, alternately for 1 mile. |
| Week 25 to 51 | Jog 1 mile, maintain pulse rate at 70% maximal, adding 100 yards per month. |
| Week 52 and over | Jog 2 miles, maintaining pulse rate at 70% maximal. |

three or four) unless the immediate postexercise pulse rate is less than 120 beats per minute.

Prior to and at the completion of the twelve-week program, the patient should be tested on the treadmill to see whether he has achieved a significant improvement in oxygen uptake. If he has not done so, he is strongly urged to make arrangements to enter the physician-supervised exercise program, either at the parent center (GBH-AMC) or a satellite center (area YMCA or community recreation center). We do not advise a postcoronary patient to begin a jogging or vigorous swimming program on his own.

### Physician-Supervised Exercise Regimen (Beginning Three Months Postcoronary Incident)

This program was originally devised for a pilot project at the Mayo Clinic by one of the authors (JDC) and Mr. Edward Koch, a physical fitness director. The program was tailored specifically for the postcoronary patient and can be modified according to the available laboratory facilities. In addition to the Mayo Clinic Study, which is in its seventh year, this exercise regimen is being used by several rehabilitation centers in Georgia, Tennessee and Florida. The fundamentals of the program are as follows:

1. Patients must be at least two months postmyocardial infarction. They must be less than sixty-five years of age. Concomitant disease such as

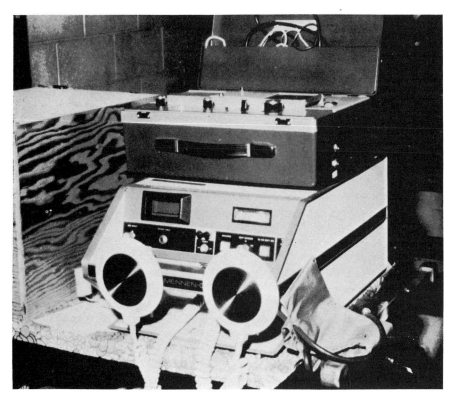

Figure 21. Resuscitation equipment for the outpatient gymnasium exercise program.

uncompensated congestive heart failure, severe hypertension (diastolic blood pressure greater than 120 mm Hg), cardiac rhythm disturbances (such as frequent PVCs, paroxysms of tachycardia), vascular disease and chronic lung disease prohibit inclusion into the program.

2. A minimum of three exercise sessions, each forty-five minutes in duration, are conducted weekly at a YMCA, local high school or community recreation center. A physician is always in attendance. Resuscitation equipment including a portable electrocardiograph machine, direct current defibrillator and emergency drug kit (Fig. 21) are on hand. The forty-five minute sessions are divided into three fifteen-minute periods. The first consists of calisthenics, the second of walk-jog activity and the third of noncompetitive group activity such as volleyball, basketball and swimming. A five-minute warm-up period and similar cool-down period is part of each session.

3. Patients are given an exercise prescription (Fig. 22) at the beginning of each week, indicating the calisthenic and walk-jog activity for that week. The prescription is based on three factors: (a) direct par-

## EXERCISE PRESCRIPTION
## GEORGIA BAPTIST HOSPITAL—ATLANTA MEDICAL CENTER
## CARDIAC REHABILITATION—GEORGIA REGIONAL
## MEDICAL PROGRAM

NAME: _____     DATE: _____

| CALISTHENICS | REPETITIONS | CALISTHENICS | REPETITIONS |
|---|---|---|---|
| Arm and shoulder | _____ | Bent leg raise | _____ |
| Toe touch | _____ | Straight leg raise | _____ |
| Knee raise | _____ | Double leg raise | _____ |
| Lateral raise | _____ | Sit-ups | _____ |
| Arm circling | _____ | Leg cross-over | _____ |
| Small jumps | _____ | | |
| | | Leg raise | _____ |
| Trunk twist | _____ | | |
| Reverse push-ups | _____ | Chest and leg raise | _____ |
| Reach and touch | _____ | Knee push-ups | _____ |

*Standing* (Arm and shoulder, Toe touch, Knee raise, Lateral raise, Arm circling)  *Sitting* (Trunk twist, Reverse push-ups, Reach and touch)  *Supine* (Bent leg raise, Straight leg raise, Double leg raise, Sit-ups, Leg cross-over)  *Side* (Leg raise)  *Prone* (Chest and leg raise, Knee push-ups)

| WALK-JOG | | GROUP ACTIVITIES | |
|---|---|---|---|
| Walk slowly _____ laps | | Volleyball | _____ |
| Walk briskly _____ laps | | Basketball | _____ |
| Jog _____ laps | | Bowling | _____ |
| | | Swimming | _____ |

SIGNED: _____ M.D.

Figure 22. Exercise photo of card for walk-jog, calisthenic and group activities.

ticipant observation by the physician in attendance, who frequently exercises with the patients; (b) preliminary and follow-up data, based on treadmill performance and oxygen consumption; and (c) the patient's subjective response to the given level of exercise (in terms of musculoskeletal side effects and respiratory effort). It is updated approximately every two weeks.

The calisthenics are conducted in five different positions and are designed to exercise the major muscle groups. Initially, the number of repetitions is low to avoid undue muscular strain and discouragement to the participant. After the initial six months, the number of repetitions are increased to the point where the individual is averaging 70 percent of his maximum pulse rate during the actual exercises. This requires radiotelemetry recording during the calisthenic period or a manual check of the pulse rate midway during each calisthenic position. The number of repetitions for a given week (for the first six months of exercise) are listed in the following chart with illustrations of each exercise as seen in Figure 23 through 39.

*Standing Position*

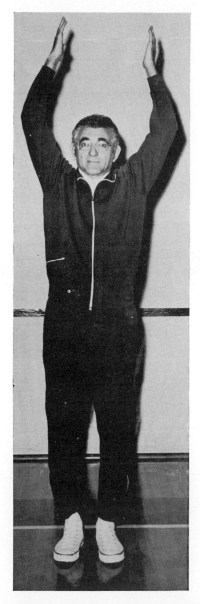

Figure 23. *Arm and shoulder loosening.* With the subject in standing position, the arms are raised overhead, bringing the palms together; the arms are then lowered to the sides, completing the sequence.

| Week | Repetitions per session | Week | Repetitions per session |
|------|------------------------|------|------------------------|
| 1 | 6 | 13 | 18 |
| 2 | 6 | 14 | 18 |
| 3 | 8 | 15 | 18 |
| 4 | 8 | 16 | 18 |
| 5 | 10 | 17 | 18 |
| 6 | 10 | 18 | 18 |
| 7 | 12 | 19 | 20 |
| 8 | 12 | 20 | 20 |
| 9 | 14 | 21 | 20 |
| 10 | 14 | 22 | 20 |
| 11 | 16 | 23 | 20 |
| 12 | 16 | 24 | 20 |

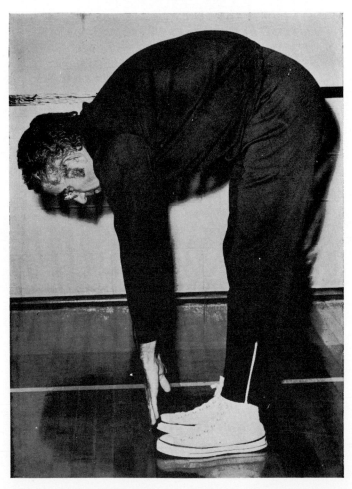

Figure 24. *Toe Touching.** Keeping the knees slightly bent, the subject flexes at the waist and touches the right fingertips to the left toes. He assumes an erect position and then touches the left fingertips to the right toes, completing the sequence.

| Week | Repetitions per session | Week | Repetitions per session |
|------|------|------|------|
| 1 | 4 | 13 | 18 |
| 2 | 4 | 14 | 18 |
| 3 | 5 | 15 | 18 |
| 4 | 5 | 16 | 18 |
| 5 | 6 | 17 | 18 |
| 6 | 6 | 18 | 18 |
| 7 | 8 | 19 | 20 |
| 8 | 8 | 20 | 20 |
| 9 | 10 | 21 | 20 |
| 10 | 10 | 22 | 20 |
| 11 | 12 | 24 | 20 |

* Omit if history of back injury.

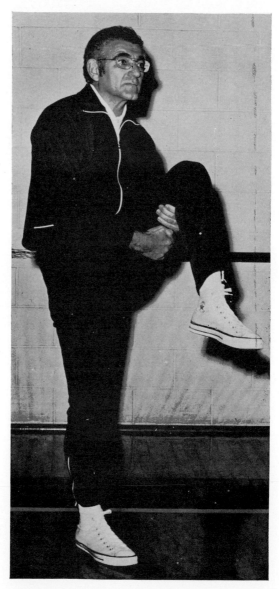

Figure 32.  *Rocking Situps.** While lying supine with hands behind the head,
        and raises it as high as he can. He then does the same thing to
        the right knee, completing one cycle.

* Omit if history of back injury.

| Week | Repetitions per session | Week | Repetitions per session |
|------|------|------|------|
| 1 | 6 | 13 | 14 |
| 2 | 6 | 14 | 14 |
| 3 | 7 | 15 | 14 |
| 4 | 7 | 16 | 14 |
| 5 | 8 | 17 | 14 |
| 6 | 8 | 18 | 14 |
| 7 | 10 | 19 | 16 |
| 8 | 10 | 20 | 16 |
| 9 | 12 | 21 | 16 |
| 10 | 12 | 22 | 16 |
| 11 | 14 | 23 | 16 |
| 12 | 14 | 24 | 16 |

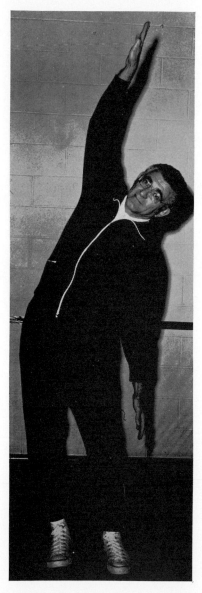

Figure 26. *Lateral Bending.* With the arms elevated in a horizontal position
        the subject bends laterally to the left, assumes an erect position,
        and then bends laterally to the right.

| Week | Repetitions per session | Week | Repetitions per session |
|------|-------------------------|------|-------------------------|
| 1    | 4                       | 13   | 12                      |
| 2    | 4                       | 14   | 12                      |
| 3    | 5                       | 15   | 12                      |
| 4    | 5                       | 16   | 12                      |
| 5    | 6                       | 17   | 12                      |
| 6    | 6                       | 18   | 12                      |
| 7    | 8                       | 19   | 14                      |
| 8    | 8                       | 20   | 14                      |
| 9    | 10                      | 21   | 14                      |
| 10   | 10                      | 22   | 14                      |
| 11   | 12                      | 23   | 14                      |
| 12   | 12                      | 24   | 14                      |

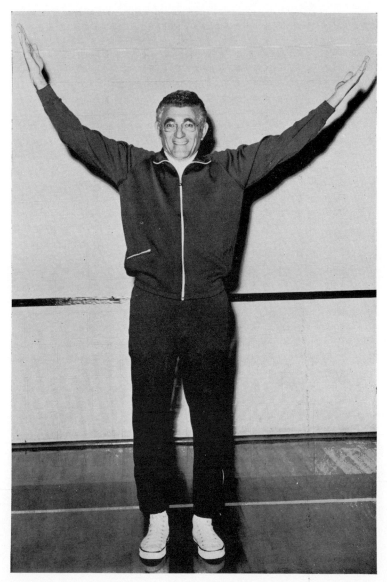

Figure 27. *Arm Circling.* The arms are elevated in a horizontal position and rotated, first clockwise, for the given number of repetitions, and then counterclockwise for the same number of times.

| Week | Repetitions per session | Week | Repetitions per session |
|------|-------------------------|------|-------------------------|
| 1  | 6  | 13 | 14 |
| 2  | 6  | 14 | 14 |
| 3  | 8  | 15 | 14 |
| 4  | 8  | 16 | 14 |
| 5  | 8  | 17 | 14 |
| 6  | 10 | 18 | 14 |
| 7  | 10 | 19 | 16 |
| 8  | 10 | 20 | 16 |
| 9  | 12 | 21 | 16 |
| 10 | 12 | 22 | 16 |
| 11 | 12 | 23 | 16 |
| 12 | 14 | 24 | 16 |

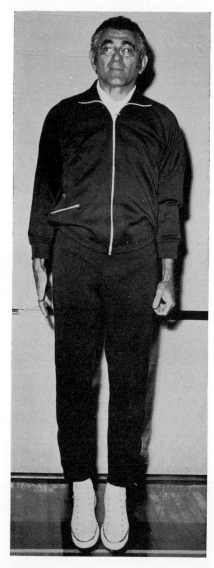

Figure 28. *Small Jumps.* The subject jumps vertically about six inches off the ground landing on the anterior aspect of the feet.

| Week | Repetitions per session | Week | Repetitions per session |
|------|------------------------|------|------------------------|
| 1 | 8 | 13 | 20 |
| 2 | 8 | 14 | 20 |
| 3 | 12 | 15 | 20 |
| 4 | 12 | 16 | 20 |
| 5 | 16 | 17 | 22 |
| 6 | 16 | 18 | 22 |
| 7 | 18 | 19 | 22 |
| 8 | 18 | 20 | 22 |
| 9 | 20 | 21 | 24 |
| 10 | 20 | 22 | 24 |
| 11 | 20 | 23 | 24 |
| 12 | 20 | 24 | 24 |

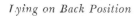

*Lying on Back Position*

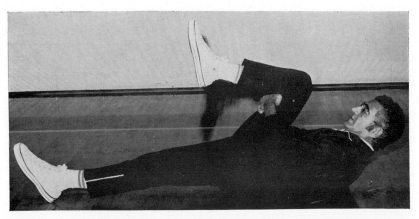

Figure 29.   *Alternate Bent Leg Raising.* While lying supine, the subject grasps
the left knee and flexes the thigh. He then repeats the maneuver
with the right knee, completing the cycle.

| *Week* | *Repetitions per session* | *Week* | *Repetitions per session* |
|---|---|---|---|
| 1 | 4 | 13 | 10 |
| 2 | 4 | 14 | 10 |
| 3 | 6 | 15 | 10 |
| 4 | 6 | 16 | 10 |
| 5 | 8 | 17 | 12 |
| 6 | 8 | 18 | 12 |
| 7 | 8 | 19 | 12 |
| 8 | 8 | 20 | 12 |
| 9 | 10 | 21 | 14 |
| 10 | 10 | 22 | 14 |
| 11 | 10 | 23 | 14 |
| 12 | 10 | 24 | 14 |

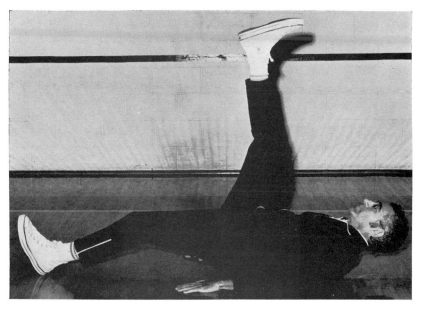

Figure 30. *Alternate Straight Leg Raising.* While lying supine the subject elevates the left leg to a forty-five-degree angle with the floor, keeping the knee straight. He repeats this with the right leg, completing one sequence.

| Week | Repetitions per session | Week | Repetitions per session |
|---|---|---|---|
| 1 | 2 | 13 | 10 |
| 2 | 2 | 14 | 10 |
| 3 | 3 | 15 | 10 |
| 4 | 4 | 16 | 10 |
| 5 | 4 | 17 | 12 |
| 6 | 4 | 18 | 12 |
| 7 | 6 | 19 | 12 |
| 8 | 6 | 20 | 12 |
| 9 | 8 | 21 | 14 |
| 10 | 8 | 22 | 14 |
| 11 | 10 | 23 | 14 |
| 12 | 10 | 24 | 14 |

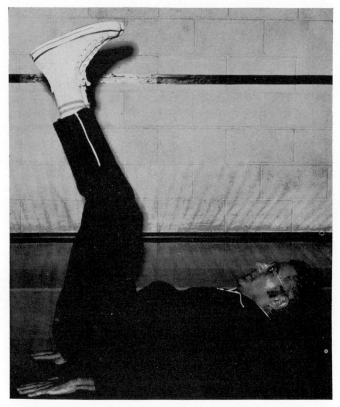

Figure 31. *Double Leg Raising and Lowering.* While lying supine the subject elevates both legs to a forty-five-degree angle with the floor, keeping the knees straight.

| Week | Repetitions per session | Week | Repetitions per session |
|---|---|---|---|
| 1 | 2 | 13 | 10 |
| 2 | 2 | 14 | 10 |
| 3 | 3 | 15 | 10 |
| 4 | 3 | 16 | 10 |
| 5 | 4 | 17 | 12 |
| 6 | 4 | 18 | 12 |
| 7 | 6 | 19 | 12 |
| 8 | 6 | 20 | 12 |
| 9 | 8 | 21 | 14 |
| 10 | 8 | 22 | 14 |
| 11 | 10 | 23 | 14 |
| 12 | 10 | 24 | 14 |

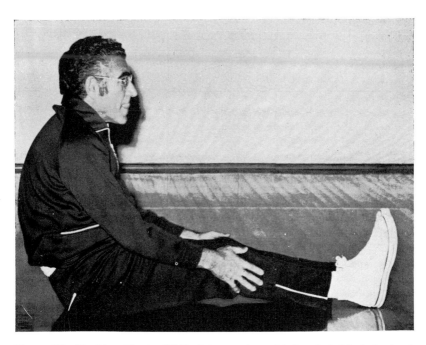

Figure 32. *Rocking Situps.* While lying supine with hands behind the head, the subject rocks to a sitting position and touches both elbows to the flexed knees.

| Week | Repetitions per session | Week | Repetitions per session |
|---|---|---|---|
| 1 | 1 | 13 | 10 |
| 2 | 2 | 14 | 10 |
| 3 | 3 | 15 | 10 |
| 4 | 3 | 16 | 10 |
| 5 | 4 | 17 | 12 |
| 6 | 4 | 18 | 12 |
| 7 | 6 | 19 | 12 |
| 8 | 6 | 20 | 12 |
| 9 | 8 | 21 | 14 |
| 10 | 8 | 22 | 14 |
| 11 | 10 | 23 | 14 |
| 12 | 10 | 24 | 14 |

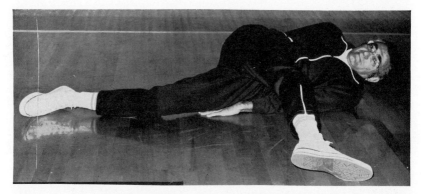

Figure 33. *Leg Crossover.* While lying supine the subject raises the right leg and touches the floor on his left with his toes. He returns to a flat position and completes one cycle by touching his left toes to the floor on his right.

| Week | Repetitions per session | Week | Repetitions per session |
|---|---|---|---|
| 1 | 1 | 13 | 6 |
| 2 | 1 | 14 | 6 |
| 3 | 2 | 15 | 6 |
| 4 | 2 | 16 | 6 |
| 5 | 3 | 17 | 8 |
| 6 | 3 | 18 | 8 |
| 7 | 4 | 19 | 8 |
| 8 | 4 | 20 | 8 |
| 9 | 5 | 21 | 10 |
| 10 | 5 | 22 | 10 |
| 11 | 6 | 23 | 10 |
| 12 | 6 | 24 | 10 |

*Side Position*

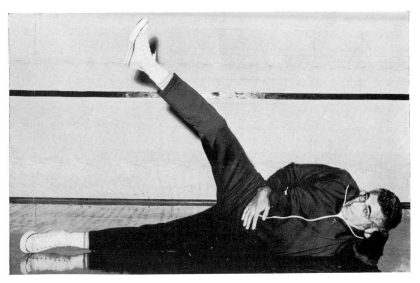

Figure 34. *Side Leg Raises.* While lying on the left side the subject raises his
right leg as high as he can for the recommended number of repetitions. He then switches to the right side and raises the left leg
the same number of times.

| Week | Repetitions per session | Week | Repetitions per session |
|------|-------------------------|------|-------------------------|
| 1 | 4 | 13 | 10 |
| 2 | 4 | 14 | 10 |
| 3 | 6 | 15 | 10 |
| 4 | 6 | 16 | 10 |
| 5 | 8 | 17 | 12 |
| 6 | 8 | 18 | 12 |
| 7 | 8 | 19 | 12 |
| 8 | 8 | 20 | 12 |
| 9 | 10 | 21 | 14 |
| 10 | 10 | 22 | 14 |
| 11 | 10 | 23 | 14 |
| 12 | 10 | 24 | 14 |

*Front (prone) Position*

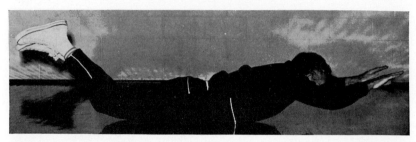

Figure 35. *Chest and Leg Raising.* Assuming a prone position the subject places the arms overhead and raises the upper part of the body and the legs as far off the ground as possible.

| Week | Repetitions per session | Week | Repetitions per session |
|---|---|---|---|
| 1 | 2 | 13 | 10 |
| 2 | 2 | 14 | 10 |
| 3 | 3 | 15 | 10 |
| 4 | 3 | 16 | 10 |
| 5 | 5 | 17 | 10 |
| 6 | 5 | 18 | 10 |
| 7 | 8 | 19 | 12 |
| 8 | 8 | 20 | 12 |
| 9 | 10 | 21 | 12 |
| 10 | 10 | 22 | 12 |
| 11 | 10 | 23 | 12 |
| 12 | 10 | 24 | 12 |

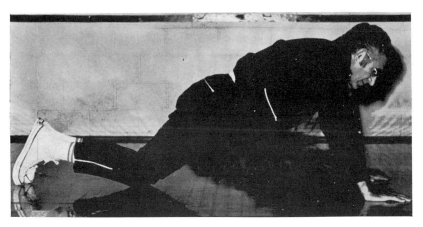

Figure 36. *Knee Pushups.* The subject positions himself on his hands and knees and touches his chest to the floor.

| Week | Repetitions per session | Week | Repetitions per session |
|---|---|---|---|
| 1 | 4 | 13 | 14 |
| 2 | 4 | 14 | 14 |
| 3 | 6 | 15 | 14 |
| 4 | 6 | 16 | 14 |
| 5 | 8 | 17 | 14 |
| 6 | 8 | 18 | 14 |
| 7 | 8 | 19 | 16 |
| 8 | 8 | 20 | 16 |
| 9 | 12 | 21 | 16 |
| 10 | 12 | 22 | 16 |
| 11 | 12 | 23 | 16 |
| 12 | 12 | 24 | 16 |

*Sitting Position*

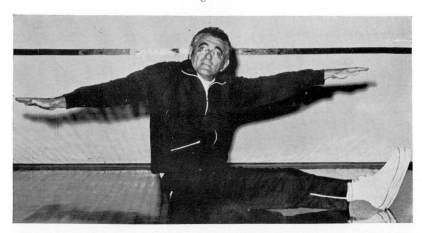

Figure 37. *Trunk Twisting.* The subject sits with legs out straight and with arms raised to a horizontal position. He twists his trunk to the left, returns to the original position, and completes one sequence by twisting the trunk to the right.

| Week | Repetitions per session | Week | Repetitions per session |
|------|------|------|------|
| 1 | 4 | 13 | 12 |
| 2 | 4 | 14 | 12 |
| 3 | 6 | 15 | 12 |
| 4 | 6 | 16 | 12 |
| 5 | 8 | 17 | 12 |
| 6 | 8 | 18 | 12 |
| 7 | 8 | 19 | 14 |
| 8 | 8 | 20 | 14 |
| 9 | 10 | 21 | 14 |
| 10 | 10 | 22 | 14 |
| 11 | 10 | 23 | 14 |
| 12 | 10 | 24 | 14 |

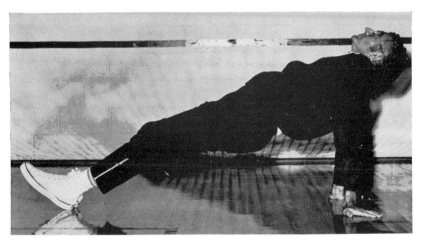

Figure 38. *Reverse Pushups.* The subject assumes a sitting position with legs out straight and hands on the floor behind his back. He pushes his body off the floor and then returns to the original position.

| Week | Repetitions per session | Week | Repetitions per session |
|------|------|------|------|
| 1 | 2 | 13 | 6 |
| 2 | 2 | 14 | 6 |
| 3 | 3 | 15 | 6 |
| 4 | 3 | 16 | 6 |
| 5 | 4 | 17 | 8 |
| 6 | 4 | 18 | 8 |
| 7 | 5 | 19 | 10 |
| 8 | 5 | 20 | 10 |
| 9 | 6 | 21 | 10 |
| 10 | 6 | 22 | 10 |
| 11 | 6 | 23 | 10 |
| 12 | 6 | 24 | 10 |

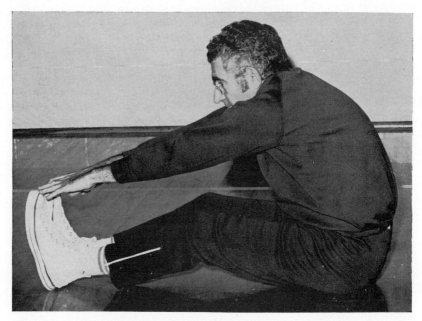

Figure 39. *Reach and Touch.* The subject assumes a sitting position with legs slightly flexed and arms at the sides. He touches the toes with his fingertips and returns to the resting position.

| Week | Repetitions per session | Week | Repetitions per session |
|---|---|---|---|
| 1 | 4 | 13 | 12 |
| 2 | 4 | 14 | 12 |
| 3 | 6 | 15 | 12 |
| 4 | 8 | 16 | 12 |
| 5 | 8 | 17 | 12 |
| 6 | 8 | 18 | 12 |
| 7 | 8 | 19 | 14 |
| 8 | 8 | 20 | 14 |
| 9 | 10 | 21 | 14 |
| 10 | 10 | 22 | 14 |
| 11 | 10 | 23 | 14 |
| 12 | 10 | 24 | 14 |

The walk-jog activity (Fig. 40) for a given week is described in Table XXIII (see page 114). The overall goal is to work up to a one-mile jog after twelve months, during which time the pulse is maintained at 70 percent of predicted maximum heart rate. A mini-

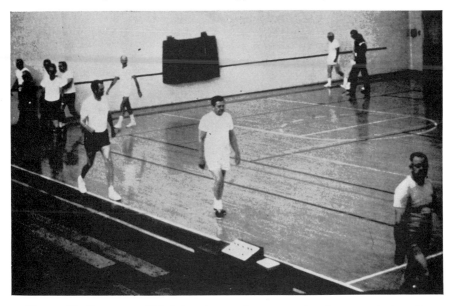

Figure 40. Postmyocardial infarction patients engaging in supervised walk-jog activities.

ature heart-monitoring instrument.* (Fig. 41) may be used initially to determine the level of exercise required to maintain this heart rate. The instrument is a battery-driven device which may be carried in a pocket or attached to the clothing. A pair of light-weight electrodes are applied to the chest and a small earphone (hearing aid type) is placed in the ear and plugged into the battery device. The device is set at the desired exercise heart rate and is switched on when exercise begins. The earphone relates the patient's own heartbeat until the target heart rate is approached, at which time the earphone remains silent as long as the pulse rate remains within a few beats of the desired rate. A warning tone is sounded when the heart rate exceeds the present rate. Patients can usually be instructed in checking their own pulse rate during interrupted jogging sessions and can thereby adjust their jogging pace with a satisfactory degree of accuracy.

*MEDRAD
4084 Mt. Royal Boulevard
Allison Park, Pa. 15101

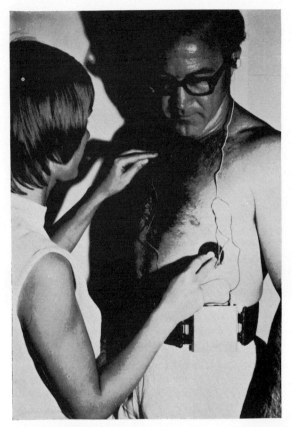

Figure 41. A subject demonstrates the use of a heart-monitoring instrument.
The battery-driven device is seen attached to the subject's belt
with lightweight electrode connections applied to the chest
wall. A small earphone is plugged into the device. Complete
explanation of the use of the device is found in the text.

If the patient misses three consecutive weeks of the program
he must undergo a repeat treadmill test and begin at the first week
level of walking and flexibility exercise. If he knows in advance
that he will be away for a week or two he may arrange to take his
exercise prescription card with him and do the walking and
calisthenic portions on his own. He is not permitted to jog.

The group activity portion is the most enjoyable to the patient,
but is potentially the most dangerous if noncompetitive rules are

not adhered to. Volleyball has been highly successful and requires no special skill for enjoyment. Basketball routines such as free throws, lay-ups, passing and full-court dribbling are also well accepted and necessitate almost constant motion. Swimming is a little harder to supervise but is an excellent form of exercise and provides a good change of pace periodically. Experienced bowlers may take advantage of the four bowling lanes and automatic pin setters in the basement of the exercise facility (Fig. 42). The blood pressure and pulse rate are determined after the patient bowls a few frames to make sure that he is tolerating the somewhat isometric activity well. For the patient with some experience in tennis or paddleball, a modified version of wall-tennis is available (Fig. 43). In the summer months the patients may exercise outdoors, provided that the resuscitation equipment can be set up nearby. Additional group activities such as badminton, ping pong, bicycle riding, darts and golf practice can be added to the regimen. Coronary-prone patients are permitted to participate in half-court basketball games at a controlled pace. The dropout rate can be minimized by providing such a wide variety of group activities. Such activities are scheduled on a rotation basis, thereby preventing overcrowding of the volleyball court and exposing indi-

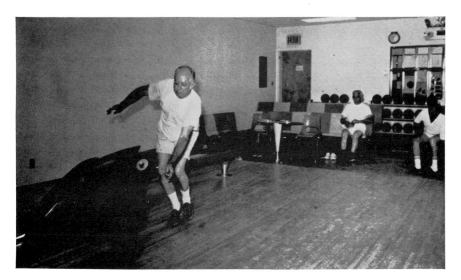

Figure 42. Postinfarction patients utilizing the gymnasium bowling lanes.

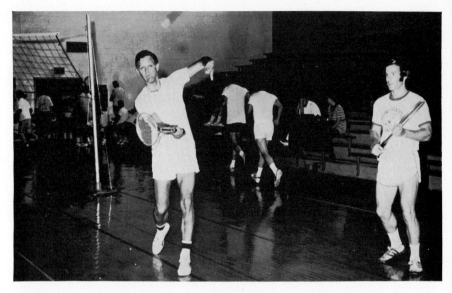

Figure 43. Patients engaging in wall tennis (using regulation tennis racquets and a rubber paddleball).

viduals to some new activities which most will find enjoyable. The physician in attendance exercises with the patients and is often the first to detect early signs of fatigue. He is always readily available to answer questions concerning any symptoms.

The progress of the exercising coronary patient can be followed in several ways. If a treadmill and equipment for oxygen consumption determination is available, this is used to determine the initial level of fitness and to record changes at two-month intervals. Using the Georgia Baptist treadmill test, an expired air sample is collected with a Douglas bag during the final minute of exercise. The resulting submaximal oxygen uptake is recorded in milliliters per kilogram per minute. In general, values below 25 are considered low, those between 30 and 40, average, and those above 40, high (Fig. 44).[278] The average initial value in Hellerstein's study [161] was 23.2 ml/kg/min. This rose to an average of 28.9 ml/kg/min. on follow-up testing. Clausen et al.[100] noted a similar increase in maximal oxygen uptake in nine patients with coronary disease who exercised regularly over a four to six-week period. If

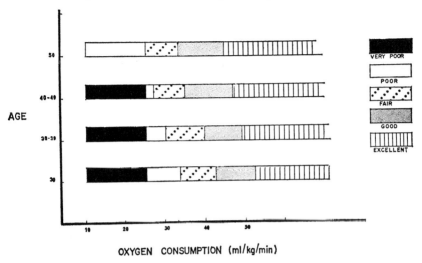

Figure 44. Graph showing physical fitness categories based on oxygen consumption and adjusted for age. Adapted from data of K. H. Cooper, M.D.

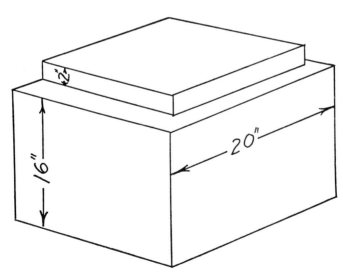

Figure 45. The bench used in the modified Harvard step test; the dimensions are specified.

a treadmill or bicycle ergometer is not available, the bench test measurement of pulse recovery (Fig. 45) is used as a rough index of the conditioning response [279] and can be easily repeated at intervals of two months. This test is a modification of the Harvard Step Test. The height of the bench is adjusted according to the patient's height (Table XXIV). It is preferable to monitor the electrocardiogram during the test in a manner previously described for the treadmill test. The individual steps up and down on the bench at a rate of thirty times per minute for a total of four minutes. At this point of fatigue, or upon completion of the test, the patient rests in a chair for one minute and then has pulse rate determinations during the first thirty seconds of each of the following three minutes. The three numbers are added together, and a pulse recovery index and fitness grade are assigned according to the scale in Table XXIV. A more elaborate step device has recently been described.[280]

Periodic screening for cardiac dysrhythmias or S-T segment depression during exercise is recommended. This can be done either by the radiotelemetry monitoring or by utilizing the paddle electrodes on the defibrillator. One of our best volleyball players was found to have significant S-T segment depression by the former method (Fig. 46). Another man was found to have asymp-

TABLE XXIV

BENCH TEST DETERMINATION OF
POSTEXERCISE PULSE RECOVERY

| Subject Height | | Bench Height |
|---|---|---|
| 5 ft. 3 in. to 5 ft. 9 in. | | 16 in. |
| 5 ft. 9 in. to 6 ft. | | 18 in. |
| over 6 ft. | | 20 in. |
| Total Pulse Counts | Recovery Index | Fitness Grade |
| > 198 | < 61 | Poor |
| 171 to 198 | 61 to 70 | Fair |
| 150 to 170 | 71 to 80 | Good |
| 133 to 149 | 81 to 90 | Very Good |
| < 133 | > 90 | Excellent |

Abbreviations: ft = feet; in = inches; total pulse count = total number of pulse beats during first 30 seconds of each of the first three minutes following exercise; > = greater; < = less than.

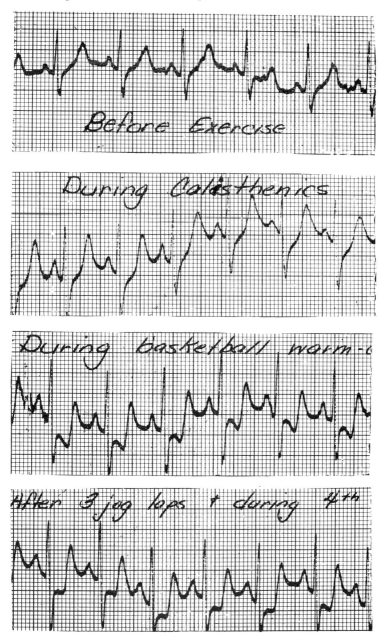

Figure 46. Telemetry-monitoring during various activities, showing S-T changes during basketball drills and walk-jog activities.

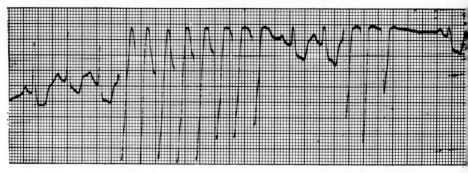

Figure 47. Asymptomatic episode of ventricular tachycardia in a fifty-seven-year-old man immediately after jogging 400 yards.

tomatic bouts of ventricular tachycardia during walk-jog activity (Fig. 47).

Charts are posted on the gym bulletin board listing the sequential results of treadmill testing, body composition analysis and blood lipid levels. The patients enjoy comparing their progress with others in the group and have shown no embarassment from such a listing.

It is unrealistic to think that all coronary patients can be reconditioned by physical training. Some patients have irreversible myocardial damage secondary to diffuse coronary atherosclerosis. If there is no improvement in treadmill performance, maximal oxygen uptake or pulse recovery (bench test) after six months of physical training, such individuals probably could be removed from the exercise program as they tend to retard the progress of other group members and increase the risk of a cardiac catastrophe during the exercise sessions. Their removal from the program should be done with considerable tactfulness and they should be encouraged to follow a daily walking program, mainly for subjective benefits.

A progress letter is sent to the referring physician at three-month intervals. Problems or situations arising in the interim that merit his attention are handled over the telephone. When the patient completes six months in the program he receives a "graduation" letter, outlining his progress in lay terms and suggesting that he enroll in one of the satellite facilities (YMCA, community centers, etc.) which is physician-approved. In order to qualify for such approval, the center must have a portable defibrillator, an emergency drug kit and allied health personnel (such as a physician's assistant or coronary care nurse) who are skilled in cardiac resuscitation.

To recapitulate, physical training is a promising new weapon in our armamentarium against coronary heart disease. The program described herein can be modified so that it can be used in a major medical center complete with sophisticated (and expensive) testing devices, or in a relatively small community hospital equipped with only an interested physician and patient. To further illustrate the chamelion-like nature of this program, let us consider the following two cases:

## Case 1

A forty-two-year-old man made an uneventful recovery from a myocardial infarction and five months later consulted his internist about physical activity. He was referred to the nearby university medical center where he underwent a complete physical examination, which included having the following laboratory tests: electrocardiogram, chest x-ray, serum cholesterol and triglycerides, two-hour postprandial blood sugar, vital capacity, MMPI and skin-fold measurements. On initial treadmill testing he progressed only to the third level, stopping because of generalized fatigue. His maximal oxygen uptake was low, being 19 ml/kg/min. He was enrolled in the previously described exercise program and progressed according to schedule for the first eight weeks, experiencing no adverse musculoskeletal side effects. Repeat testing revealed that he was able to complete the fourth level of treadmill elevation. The oxygen uptake was now 24 ml/kg/min. As he began the ninth week of exercise, a cardiopacer was used to regulate his jogging pace at that necessary to maintain a pulse rate of 135 beats/minute. This pace was well tolerated by the patient. Radiotelemetry revealed no S-T segment depression or arrhythmias.

## Case 2

A forty-nine-year-old man had been admitted to a small community hospital (eighty beds) for evaluation of severe angina pectoris. His physical examination was unremarkable, and there were no abnormalities in serum lipids or in glucose tolerance. He was advised to stop cigarette smoking and was on a combination of isosorbide dinitrate and propranolol. Despite maximum doses of the latter, he continued to require an average of fifteen nitroglycerine tablets daily and was unable to hold a job. Coronary arteriograms revealed a 75 percent narrowing of the left anterior descending coronary artery and a 60 percent occlusion of the right circumflex coronary. The patient was enrolled in a physical training program at the local YMCA. The group was small, numbering only four men, and was supervised by a physical director and a physician. Initially he was given a Master's test (which was positive) and found to have a pulse recovery index (Table XXIV) of sixty, which was poor. Although initially quite apprehensive during the exercise sessions, he had no difficulty in following the weekly exercise prescription. At two-month intervals he had follow-up Master's 2-Step and pulse recovery testing; the former remained positive, although the S-T segment depression was reduced from 2 to 1 mm, while the pulse recovery index was now 75, which was indicative of a good response. With a little practice the patient was able to measure his radial pulse rate during interrupted jogging and adjusted his pace to maintain an average pulse rate of 135 beats/minute. He was able to return to work but still required approximately five nitroglycerine tablets per day.

*Chapter X*

# DISADVANTAGES AND
# COMPLICATIONS OF EXERCISE

THE TRUE DISADVANTAGES of exercise with regards to long-term effects are less well supported than the advantages. In 1966, Keys reported in European population sample studies that the more physically active Finns have more coronary deaths than do American whites. Other similar studies [281] have shown little or no difference in coronary heart disease death rates among various occupations involving different levels of physical activity in the Chicago area. Although few studies relate obvious disadvantages of exercise, there have been to date no statistically significant control studies to show that exercise is definitely advantageous in the management of coronary heart disease. This lack of positive evidence has been a limiting factor in establishing the role of exercise in the therapeutic program in many of our less progressive medical centers.

Complications of exercise can be subdivided into two groups, i.e., *cardiac* and *noncardiac*.

## Cardiac Complications

Regarding *cardiac* complications, the major factors to be concerned with are sudden death, myocardial infarction and arrhythmias. Fox and Haskell [282] have reported that certain changes in physical activity may be instrumental in patients with myocardial infarction. On occasions the news media report the occurrence of sudden unexpected death in a subject while jogging; not infrequently, we hear authenticated verbal reports of such complications. These deaths are most likely due to myocardial infarction, arrhythmias or cerebral vascular accidents.

With regard to myocardial infarction, we have seen a typical example [283] in a forty-four-year-old white insurance salesman who was hospitalized at the University Hospital of San Diego County complaining of severe chest pain which had developed while he was jogging in a "Run for your Life" exercise class. He had previously been well, although he had not actively exercised in over twenty years. He had smoked two packs of cigarettes per day, had been moderately overweight all his adult life, and recently had consumed alcoholic beverages in moderate to heavy amounts. His father died at forty-two years of age from an acute myocardial infarction. Prior to entering the exercise program, the patient obtained the recommended blood pressure, heart rate and cholesterol levels from his private physician. An electrocardiogram was not taken. In the exercise program, he had been started in Plan B of Bowerman and Harris,[143] which is a program for individuals in average physical condition. After three weeks he had not lost his initial muscle soreness. On the day of admission, while attempting to jog one and a half miles, he was unable to keep up with the others in his group of ten. Finally, he alternated walking and jogging, fifty steps each, and then jogged almost one mile, after which he noted severe substernal chest pain associated with dyspnea and diaphoresis.

On physical examination he was moderately obese but normotensive. Results of cardiopulmonary examination were normal and no other pertinent physical findings were noted. Initial laboratory data included a normal x-ray film of the chest and normal cholesterol and blood glucose levels. Serial electrocardiograms showed changes of an acute inferior wall myocardial infarction (Fig. 48). Results of enzyme determinations supported this diagnosis. The hospital course was uneventful and the patient was discharged at the end of the third week.

An example of an apparent dysrhythmia has been seen in a fifty-one-year-old man who had entered a running program following a physical examination which showed no abnormalities. He had noted malaise and fatigue two days before admission and chest pain on the right side posteriorly, that persisted throughout the day of admission. Despite the latter, he played volleyball for forty-five minutes and ran one lap (440 yards). On completion of the latter he suddenly collapsed and a physician running behind him found him to be cyanotic, unresponsive, pulseless and with fixed dilated

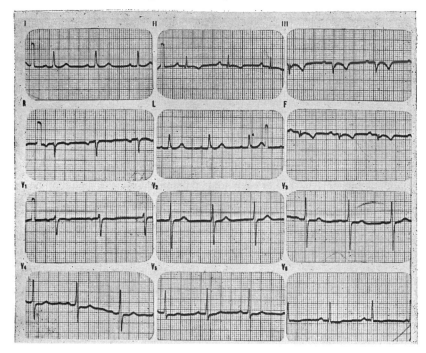

Figure 48. Twelve lead electrocardiogram of a forty-four-year-old male who had an acute inferior myocardial infarction while jogging. The abnormal Q-waves and ST-T segments are seen in leads II, III and F.

pupils. He was successfully resuscitated in three minutes and hospitalized thirty minutes later. Family history was significant in that his father had died suddenly at forty-eight years of age. A brother had an initial myocardial infarction at the age of thirty-two and died from another at the age of thirty-eight. Another brother died at the age of fifty-eight of a "heart attack", and a third brother was hospitalized for several myocardial infarctions in his early fifties.

Results of physical examination on arrival at the hospital showed a blood pressure of 180/100 mm Hg. Other than a grade 1/6 early systolic murmur at the apex, findings from the cardiovascular examination were unremarkable. The white blood cell count was 6,400/cu mm with a normal differential count. The hemoglobin level was 14.1 gm/100 cc. The initial serum lactic dehydrogenase value was fourteen units on admission and a week later, two units. The level of serum glutamic oxaloacetic transaminase drawn three days after admission was normal.

The aforementioned cases and our gymnasium program results serve to suggest that complete screening of patients is of importance. Although it is appreciated that screening may not have detected the presence of coronary atherosclerotic disease in either of the cases reported, it is also probable that if high risk individuals were detected, such complications might be avoided.

As explained in other sections, it is truly felt that a detailed search for coronary risk factors should be undertaken prior to commencement of an exercise program.[284] Symptoms of chest discomfort, current medications, cigarette and alcohol consumption, previous exercise history, familial tendency toward coronary disease and history of hypertension and diabetes mellitus should all be discussed. The physical examination should place emphasis on blood pressure, heart rate, cardiac murmurs, weight and evidence of atherogenesis (such as xanthomas). Other screening laboratory work, such as exercise testing and blood studies are suggested and will be discussed in Chapter XI. During training, patients should be repeatedly warned not to exercise if they have recently noted ill health or experienced chest discomfort.

### *Noncardiac Complications*

The noncardiac complications of exercise tend to debilitate the exercise enthusiast and cause dropouts from exercise programs. Such problems—usually involving the musculoskeletal system— are not infrequently seen. Harris and Bowerman [143] reported seven subjects who developed acute gout in a group of 265 subjects who were involved in an exercise program. Other reported complications include development of petechiae,[285] joggers heel,[286] exacerbations of osteoarthritis,[287] and severe, persistent muscular soreness which accounted for thirty-four of the ninety-eight dropouts reported by Harris and Bowerman.[143] In addition, one of the authors (JDC) has observed Achilles tendonitis and a march fracture directly related to jogging.

In a postmyocardial infarction gym exercise program (described

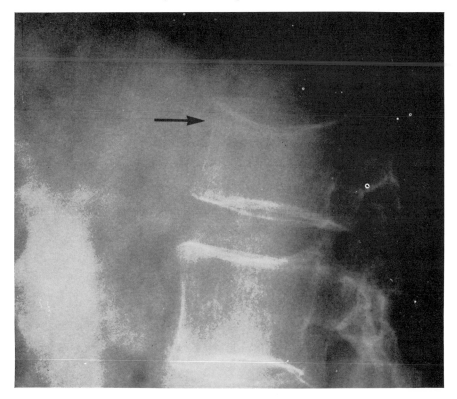

Figure 49. X-ray films of lumbosacral spine showing compression fracture as noted by arrow.

in detail in Chapter XI), we have seen a number of minor but notable problems. These include ecchymoses, sprained fingers (secondary to volleyball), muscular strains, aggravation of pseudogout, aggravation of previous knee injuries (cartilage or ligaments) and an occasional minor laceration. The most debilitating noncardiac complication occurring in our program has been that of a sixty-one-year-old man who fell in the "seated position" while playing volleyball. He suffered a compression fracture of the lumbar spine; x-ray changes are seen in Figure 49. He was treated conservatively and has subsequently returned to the program.

It is clear, therefore, that exercise programs for patients with coronary heart disease are, at times, interrupted by cardiac and noncardiac complications. These complications may delay the patient's progress in training, but do not necessarily cause termination of his participation in the program. Further comments on the prevention of such complications and ways to make physical training more practical and efficient are forthcoming.

*Chapter XI*

# AN OUTPATIENT GYM EXERCISE PROGRAM
# FOR PATIENTS WITH RECENT MYOCARDIAL
# INFARCTION AT GEORGIA BAPTIST HOSPITAL

A NUMBER OF CLINICAL STUDIES [27,29,74,75,76,288,289] from several
countries emphasize the benefit of organized physical activity
programs in patients with coronary heart disease and recent myocardial infarction. Although many of the known subjects with
recent myocardial infarction are not incorporated into such programs, such management is becoming more popular among
physicians as the feasibility and safety of these programs becomes
more apparent and more patients become motivated. The purpose
of this chapter is to present the method of evaluation and training
used and the preliminary results of an outpatient exercise program
for patients with recent myocardial infarction who were trained in
the gymnasium of a large metropolitan community hospital.

Patients were evaluated for the exercise phase of the cardiac
rehabilitation program after receipt of a written clinical summary
of hospitalization and referral from their individual private physicians. They were at least ten weeks postmyocardial infarction.
No one was admitted to the program if he had persistent complicating dysrhythmias, heart failure, evidence of ventricular dysfunction, or a complicating systemic illness such as uncontrolled
diabetes mellitus or obstructive lung disease. Angina pectoris was
not considered a disqualifying complication. Some patients were
receiving antianginal medications such as nitrates and beta block-
ing agents that could affect exercise performance. However, there
was no change of medications during the program (between testing periods) except for less frequent use of short-acting nitrates in
several patients. Candidates for the program were evaluated by the
team of physicians, physician's assistants and nurses in charge of the
rehabilitation program. At this time a brief history and physical
examination (including careful cardiac palpation and ausculta-

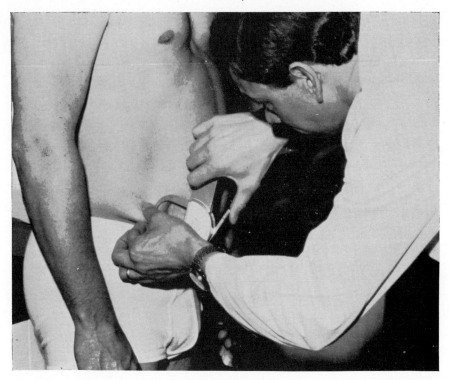

Figure 50. The technique of skin fold measurement is demonstrated. The instrument utilized is the Lange skin fold caliper.

tion) were done. Emphasis was placed on a coronary risk factor profile to include history of hypertension, smoking and family history of coronary disease. The mechanics and purpose of the exercise program and testing were explained to the patient and his family. The subjects were submitted to a baseline resting electrocardiogram which was reviewed by the physician, followed by a submaximal treadmill exercise test (as a measure of exercise capacity) with oxygen consumption studies at rest and with exercise. Patients on medications continued these during their testing periods. The method of exercise testing involving a motor-driven treadmill at a constant speed of two miles per hour with incremental elevation of the slope has been described elsewhere. Additional evaluation included body weight, skin fold measurements (Fig. 50), and abdominal, chest and thigh circumferences. The mechanics and purpose of the exercise program were explained to the patient and his family.

The patient was then scheduled for the second part of his evaluation for the exercise program, to be done one day later. At this time, the Bench test, (a simple step test) was performed. This was done in order to have a simple exercise evaluation that can be done in any physician's office to compare with the more elaborate treadmill test. Spirometry for evaluation of pulmonary function and blood studies for lipid profile (including serum cholesterol and triglyceride determination) were also performed. SMA-12 determinations were done to include glucose and uric acid levels. All blood studies were done in the fasting state—twelve hours after the last meal. At this visit (ten to twelve weeks after myocardial infarction), the patient was informed of his official acceptance into the program (unless the evaluation revealed some of the aforementioned complications that required further evaluation by the private physician), and any further questions regarding the program were answered by the staff for him or his family. At the final part of the second evaluation, the subject was given a tour of the hospital gymnasium facility.

The gymnasium utilized in the program is a 19,500-square-foot building which houses a full-size basketball court which is also utilized as a volleyball court. The view of the hospital facilities in Figure 51 shows the gym and its relation to the hospital. There are spectator stands adjacent to the volleyball court with a seating capacity of 500 persons. A thirty by thirty-foot swimming pool, ping pong area (two tables), a four lane bowling alley and areas for shuffleboard and indoor horseshoes are also utilized. The exercise sequence for the subjects involves classes on Monday, Wednesday and Friday (forty-five minutes per class). A class meets at 3:30 PM, 4:15 PM and 5:00 PM on each of these days. Each session is divided into a fifteen-minute period each of walk-jog sequence, calisthenics and team sports—usually volleyball; the specifics of each of these periods is described elsewhere as is the walk-jog sequence. The sequence serves only as a guideline and is modified individually according to the subject's submaximal treadmill exercise test performance. The level of exercise in each of these categories is prescribed by individual prescription for each patient by

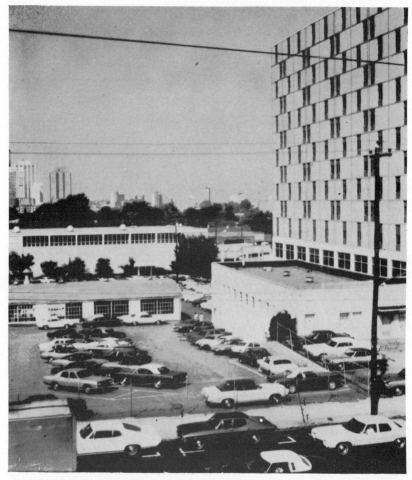

Figure 51. The gymnasium is shown in the middle-left of the photo (several large shrubs in front) as it relates to the hospital facility (tallest building on the right). The metropolitan skyline of Atlanta is seen in the background.

the program director or his associate based on the initial work load attained in testing heart rate, blood pressure and S-T segment response. Prescriptions are altered and increased according to the subject's exercise heart rate, longevity in the program and rate of conditioning. At each session the nurse or technologist checks and records the patient's resting blood pressure by cuff sphygmo-

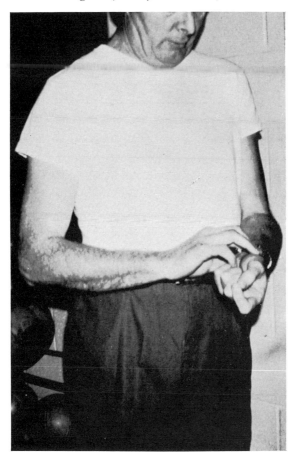

Figure 52. Patient is shown checking heart rate after an exercise sequence by palpation of the radial pulse.

manometer. At this time the physician, nurse, physician's assistant or technologist has the opportunity to converse briefly with the patient in order to detect any obvious acute emotional or physical change; specific note is made of symptoms of chest discomfort, dizziness, faintness or palpitation, and the daily exercise may be decreased accordingly. The patient himself then checks and records his own heart rate by radial or carotid palpation before and after each fifteen-minute exercise period (See Fig. 52).

In addition to medical personnel trained in cardiopulmonary

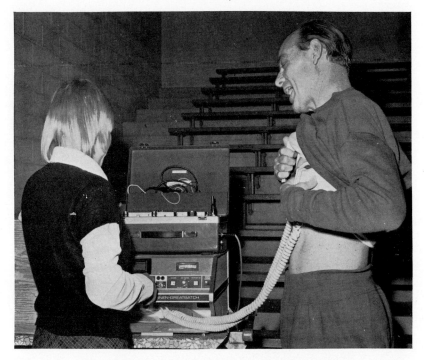

Figure 53. Nurse coordinator shown recording "instant" electrocardiographic rhythm strip on patient prior to walk-jog sequence. The signal is transmitted through the defibrillator paddles to the graphic recorder.

resuscitation, the gym is equipped with closed circuit television monitoring from the swimming pool, ping pong area and volleyball court with a central receiving set in the gym office. Cardiopulmonary resuscitation equipment (including airway, defibrillator, electrocardiogram machine and ambu bag) as well as cardiac drugs are located on an emergency cart. Both a litter and a wheel chair are available in the gym for patient transportation to the hospital emergency room, which is only a five-minute walk from the gym and employs a direct telephone extension. Instant electrocardiogram rhythm strips are available through recorded signals via defibrillator paddles as seen in Figure 53.

All patients admitted to the program understand that they are to have repeat testing (identical to that on entering the program) at three-month intervals for at least six months. The subjects are also given instruction in coronary risk factor modification and, as their study results return, if indicated, they are given private or group instruction on dietary modification for the purpose of alleviating coronary risk factors such as smoking, abnormal lipid patterns and control of hypertension. Educational conferences are also held weekly for the patients and their families by physicians, nurses, dietitians, social workers and chaplains.

At the six-month point in the program, the subjects are given the privilege of continuing in the hospital program or are given an exercise prescription by which to continue their individual program at home or at some other facility. After the six-month testing patients are submitted to the submaximal treadmill test only every six months as a method of follow-up evaluation. At the end of the three-month and the six-month testing periods, the patient's private physician receives a written progress report.

From January, 1971, through August, 1972, seventy-three patients were enrolled in the exercise program after having qualified through evaluation and testing. No control group has thus far been utilized. Of these seventy-three enrolled, sixty-seven are male and six are female subjects, all of whom are white. The lack of black patients is notable; however, this is explained by the fact that only two eligible blacks have been referred thus far; one of these lived too far from the exercise facility to attend, and the other was not sufficiently motivated to complete the testing and enter the program. No black subjects were rejected. The age range was from thirty-six to seventy-two years with a mean age of 54.4 years. Thirty-two subjects had anterior myocardial infarctions by electrocardiograms, thirty had inferior and eleven subendocardial. Forty-two patients have completed three months of the training program and, of these, twenty-two have completed six months with an overall average of 75 percent attendance. Twenty-one subjects have completed less than three months of training and seven dropped out of the program before completion of three months. Of the seven dropouts, five gave as reasons their busy work schedule and two had medical reasons; the two medical reasons were recurrent refractory angina pectoris in one and a cerebral vascular accident in the other.

# INCREASE IN TREADMILL TEST TIME
# IN MINUTES

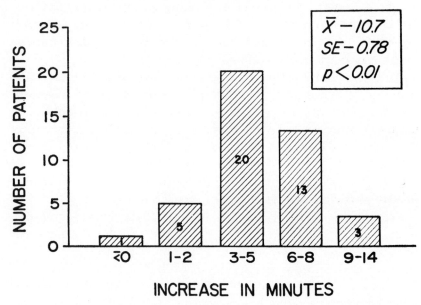

Figure 54. Bar graph showing the change in submaximal treadmill test time for the forty-two patients at the three-month retesting point in the exercise training program. Mean value, confidence limits and significance are noted.

Of the forty-two patients (those who completed three months or more of training) one had no change in repeat (three-month) submaximal treadmill exercise test (STET) time (for the same heart rate end point as in initial testing, anginal pain or positive test for ischemic heart disease), five had increased their STET by one to two minutes, twenty by three to five minutes, thirteen by six to eight minutes and three by nine to fourteen minutes. The mean increase in STET time for all forty-two patients was 10.7 minutes and was statistically significant (p<.01). These changes are illustrated in Figure 54. Ten of these forty-two patients were smokers at the time of exercise testing but none had smoked within the hour prior to testing.

# RESTING SYSTOLIC BLOOD PRESSURE

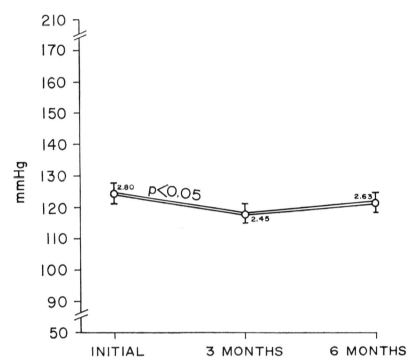

Figure 55. Figure showing the mean resting systolic blood pressure for all forty-two patients at the initial, three-month and six-month period of the exercise program. Mean values for blood pressure, confidence limits and significance are noted.

On retesting, the systemic arterial pressure decreased by at least 8 mm Hg systolic and 4 mm Hg diastolic in twenty-three subjects at rest and twenty-four subjects during peak exercise. The mean resting systolic blood pressure for all forty-two patients decreased from 124.4 mm Hg initially to 117.9 mm Hg at the three-month follow-up testing period. This is statistically significant (p<.05) (See Figs. 55 and 56).

The resting heart rate decreased by five beats per minute in twenty-five of forty-two patients (60%), did not change in eleven of forty-two patients (26%) and increased by five beats per minute in nine of forty-two patients (21%). The mean resting heart rate

# PEAK SYSTOLIC BLOOD PRESSURES

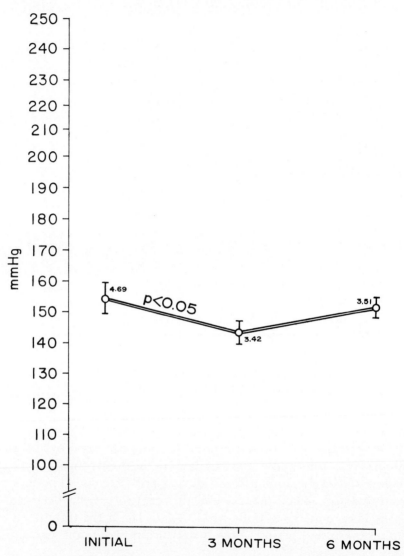

Figure 56. Figure showing the mean exercise blood pressure for all forty-two patients at the initial, three-month and six-month period of the exercise program. Mean value for blood pressure, confidence limits and significance are noted.

# RESTING HEART RATES

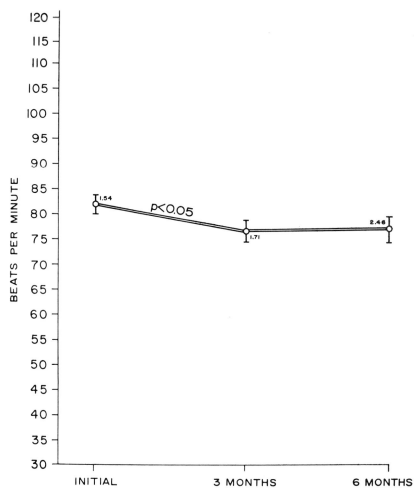

Figure 57. Figure showing the mean resting heart rate for all forty-two patients at the initial, three-month and six-month period of the exercise program. Mean values for heart rate, confidence limits and significance are noted.

for all patients decreased from 82.3 beats per minute initially to 77.2 beats per minute at the three-month follow-up testing period and was statistically significant (p<.05) (See Fig. 57). Recovery

## EXERCISE  QUOTIENTS

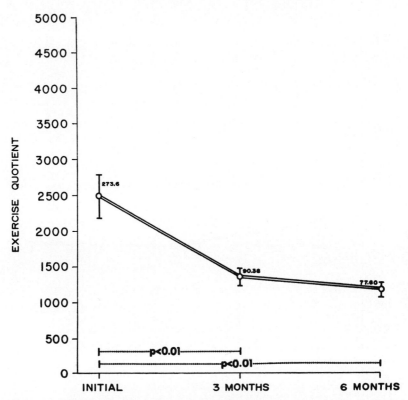

Figure 58. Figure showing the exercise quotient for all patients at the initial three-month and six-month testing periods. Mean values,
confidence limits and significance are noted.

heart rate analysis in retesting at three months revealed that at
one-minute recovery, twenty of forty-two (48 percent of the subjects), at two-minute recovery, sixteen (38 percent), and at three-
minute recovery twenty-one (50 percent) decreased their heart
rate by five beats per minute or more.

As an index of cardiac performance the exercise quotient (Eq),
(peak heart rate in beats per minute times the peak systolic blood
pressure in millimeters of mercury divided by STET time in
minutes) decreased in all but one of the patients. The mean Eq
for all patients decreased from 2500.8 initially to 1370.9 at three-

month testing and to 1221.6 at six-month testing. This was statistically significant, both from initial testing to three months (p<.01) and from initial compared to six months (p<.01) (See Fig. 58).

Only three patients had positive electrocardiographic evidence for ischemic heart disease on initial STET. Two of these had negative tests after three months. Several patients on antianginal medication required less short-acting medication as they progressed in the exercise program.

Of the forty-two patients completing three or more months of the program, all but four are gainfully employed. Of the seven subjects dropping out of the program before the end of three months of training, one had worsening of his Eq as well as a decreased repeat STET time; of the other six, three improved their Eq, one did not change his STET time, and three had no follow-up testing.

Several patients remaining in the program had minor injuries such as soft tissue ecchymoses, "pulled" hamstrings, sprained ankles and generalized muscular soreness that caused temporary cessation of their activity. All of these, however, returned to the program without consequence.

Regarding body weight and fasting blood chemistry and blood lipid studies, no specific patterns or correlations have evolved. Of the forty-two patients, twenty (47%) had a decrease in weight of at least four pounds or more. Twenty-five (60%) had decrease in serum cholesterol of 20 mgm% or more, twenty-two (52%) had a decrease in serum triglycerides of 15 mgm% or more and twenty (47%) had a decrease of 0.3 mgm% or more in serum uric acid. In twelve of the total forty-two, both cholesterol and triglycerides were decreased. For twenty-two patients reviewed at the six-month follow-up period a statistically significant mean weight decrease (p<.01) of 175.1 pounds to 162.7 pounds was recorded. For the sixteen patients who had repeat triglyceride determination at the six-month follow-up period, there was a mean decrease from 190.4 mgm% to 143.8 mgm% which was also statistically significant (p<.01). Table XXV shows the specific data for each of the patients.

All patients remaining in the program for at least three months (forty-two at this point) expressed the fact that they enjoyed the

TABLE XXV

SUMMARY OF DATA ON EXERCISING PATIENTS WITH RECENT MYOCARDIAL INFARCTION

| Pt. # | Weight in lbs. | | | Serum Cholesterol mgm% | | | Serum Triglycerides mgm% | | | Serum Uric Acid mgm% | | | Change in STET time in min. | |
|---|---|---|---|---|---|---|---|---|---|---|---|---|---|---|
| | Initial | 3 mo. | 6 mo. | Initial | 3 mo. | 6 mo. | Initial | 3 mo. | 6 mo. | Initial | 3 mo. | 6 mo. | 3 mo. | 6 mo. |
| 1 | 175 | 175 | 168 | 225 | NT | NT | 116 | NT | NT | 6.6 | NT | NT | 14 | 0 |
| 2 | 167 | 165 | 165 | 221 | NT | NT | 176 | NT | NT | NT | NT | NT | 3 | 3 |
| 3 | 173 | 173 | 173 | 247 | NT | NT | 135 | NT | NT | 8.2 | NT | NT | 2 | -1 |
| 4 | 158 | 147 | 146 | 265 | 274 | NT | 440 | 350 | NT | 7.7 | 6.3 | NT | 5 | 4 |
| 5 | 180 | 190 | 185 | 208 | NT | NT | 55 | NT | NT | NT | NT | NT | 5 | 0 |
| 6 | 165 | 170 | 174 | 275 | 300 | 256 | 103 | 70 | 92 | 7.4 | 5.9 | 5.8 | 3 | 3 |
| 7 | 150 | 150 | 152 | 237 | 254 | 277 | 225 | 130 | 155 | 6.5 | 8.5 | 7.8 | 5 | 6 |
| 8 | 178 | 172 | 173 | 266 | 295 | 290 | 285 | 189 | 180 | 8.2 | 7.7 | 6.1 | 3 | -3 |
| 9 | 196 | 195 | 192 | 252 | 203 | 195 | 165 | 134 | 150 | 8.0 | 8.9 | 7.6 | 3 | -1 |
| 10 | 180 | 170 | 165 | 220 | 247 | 229 | 217 | 115 | 70 | 7.4 | 6.6 | 6.1 | 7 | 1 |
| 11 | 151 | 150 | 150 | 190 | 172 | 246 | 195 | 140 | NT | 6.2 | 5.9 | 6.4 | 3 | 8.5 |
| 12 | 169 | 171 | 173 | 215 | 210 | 221 | 98 | 92 | 126 | 7.3 | 7.0 | 6.6 | 5 | 2.5 |
| 13 | 172 | 176 | 171 | 305 | 275 | 295 | 210 | 168 | 195 | 7.5 | 6.8 | 6.8 | 6 | 6 |
| 14 | 167 | 169 | 170 | 232 | 220 | 234 | 110 | 110 | 123 | 6.9 | 6.1 | 6.2 | 1 | 3 |
| 15 | 186 | 189 | 185 | 316 | 295 | 355 | 180 | 181 | 243 | 8.4 | 8.5 | 8.7 | 7 | 3 |
| 16 | 126 | 125 | 130 | 197 | 205 | 185 | 160 | 170 | 115 | 6.7 | 7.2 | 7.1 | 4 | 3 |
| 17 | 160 | 174 | 175 | 295 | 276 | 271 | 130 | 162 | 139 | 5.0 | 4.8 | 6.0 | -1 | 3 |
| 18 | 153 | 143 | 142 | 256 | 268 | 263 | 75 | 135 | 135 | 4.0 | 4.6 | 4.9 | 6 | 6 |
| 19 | 158 | 155 | 147 | 393 | 400 | 345 | 215 | 100 | 116 | 5.1 | 5.2 | 4.8 | 5 | 1 |
| 20 | 123 | 130 | 124 | 203 | 258 | 256 | 135 | 195 | 160 | 3.5 | 4.0 | 4.1 | 1 | -4 |
| 21 | 167 | 157 | 155 | 246 | 288 | 260 | 150 | 138 | 158 | 4.4 | 5.4 | 4.9 | 4 | 5 |
| 22 | 179 | 177 | 175 | 305 | 337 | 310 | 115 | 255 | 216 | 5.6 | 8.6 | 6.7 | 3 | 4 |
| 23 | 239 | 227 | NT | 208 | 190 | NT | 119 | 90 | NT | 6.5 | 7.3 | NT | 10 | 0 |
| 24 | 207 | 207 | NT | 265 | 281 | NT | 260 | 315 | NT | 6.0 | 6.9 | NT | 8 | NT |

| | | | | | | | | | | | | | |
|---|---|---|---|---|---|---|---|---|---|---|---|---|---|
| 25 | 190 | 184 | NT | 271 | 240 | NT | 298 | 330 | NT | 8.1 | 9.0 | NT | 4 | NT |
| 26 | 198 | 192 | NT | 215 | 175 | NT | 98 | 75 | NT | 6.4 | 6.0 | NT | 6 | NT |
| 27 | 188 | 190 | NT | 210 | 185 | NT | 105 | 125 | NT | 5.0 | 4.7 | NT | 2 | NT |
| 28 | 143 | 141 | NT | 261 | 250 | NT | 130 | 110 | NT | 5.3 | 6.9 | NT | 3 | NT |
| 29 | 188 | 192 | NT | 221 | 215 | NT | 393 | 335 | NT | 7.1 | 7.2 | NT | 4 | NT |
| 30 | 170 | 165 | NT | 300 | 319 | NT | 340 | 436 | NT | 6.5 | 6.5 | NT | 6 | NT |
| 31 | 190 | 185 | NT | 201 | 191 | NT | 58 | 93 | NT | 6.4 | 7.2 | NT | 8 | NT |
| 32 | 195 | 184 | NT | 266 | 255 | NT | 185 | 266 | NT | 9.5 | 9.2 | NT | 11 | NT |
| 33 | 193 | 200 | NT | 271 | 265 | NT | 117 | 104 | NT | 7.3 | 7.2 | NT | 7 | NT |
| 34 | 164 | 160 | NT | 340 | 240 | NT | 185 | 125 | NT | 6.7 | 6.9 | NT | 6 | NT |
| 35 | 170 | 165 | NT | 239 | 192 | NT | 213 | 150 | NT | 5.3 | 4.1 | NT | 7 | NT |
| 36 | 176 | 171 | NT | 200 | 186 | NT | 143 | 70 | NT | 6.4 | 5.5 | NT | 8 | NT |
| 37 | 193 | 194 | NT | 196 | 196 | NT | 158 | 155 | NT | 6.6 | 6.9 | NT | 4 | NT |
| 38 | 190 | 188 | NT | 255 | 285 | NT | 625 | 655 | NT | 6.3 | 6.0 | NT | 3 | NT |
| 39 | 156 | 160 | NT | 280 | 249 | NT | 110 | 108 | NT | 7.8 | 6.5 | NT | 8 | NT |
| 40 | 170 | 165 | NT | 274 | 271 | NT | 175 | 209 | NT | 8.9 | 9.7 | NT | 1 | NT |
| 41 | 185 | 185 | NT | 335 | 324 | NT | 405 | 78 | NT | 5.8 | 5.7 | NT | 5 | NT |
| 42 | 181 | 179 | NT | 201 | 217 | NT | 299 | 238 | NT | 6.0 | 3.3 | NT | 5 | NT |

mo. = months
lbs. = pounds
– = minus
# = number

mgm% = milligrams percent
STET = submaximal treadmill exercise test
NT = not tested

program and felt it was beneficial. They felt that tensions were relieved, that they felt better and were acquiring confidence in their ability to perform physical tasks during the exercise classes and in their daily activity at work and at home.

Although no control group has been studied, the results of our program at this time are consistent in some ways, but not so in others, with the aforementioned reported studies.[27,29,74,75,76,288,289] The increase in STET time (as a measure of exercise capacity) from baseline to the three-month follow-up from three to eight minutes (Fig. 54) in thirty-three of the forty-two patients reflects notable improvement in the time endured on the constant speed (2 mph), variable grade test, and the significant change in the mean values from initial to three-month follow-up testing is supportive. Although some degree of this improvement may be related to more familiarity with the testing techniques (not seen in dropouts), it is felt that the greater increases in time reflect benefits from training. With regard to blood pressure change, twenty-three of forty-two (55%) patients decreased their pressure at rest and the mean value decrease for all forty-two patients from initial to three-month follow-up testing was statistically significant (p<.05). Twenty-four of forty-two patients (57%) decreased their blood pressure with peak exercise and the mean value for all patients decreased significantly (with peak exercise) from the initial to the three-month follow-up testing (p<.05). Twenty-seven of forty-two patients (52%) decreased their blood pressure at two minutes postexercise. Whereas these alterations are not too impressive, the fact that greater than 50 percent of all forty-two patients lowered their resting blood pressure is notable. Statistically significant changes in mean values at rest and peak exercise are also notable, even with the small number of total patients.

More impressive was the data on change in resting heart rate in which twenty-five of the forty-two patients (60%) decreased their rate by five beats per minute, and the mean value decrease for all patients was statistically significant (p<.05). This is consistent with the results of Frick *et al.*[29] and Morgan *et al.*[289] Of nine patients (21%) who had an increase in resting heart rate after three months of training, two had a history of severe myocardial infarction and were felt to have considerable residual cardiac damage;

three had recurrences of angina pectoris during the training period, were limited in their progress and felt not to be as well-trained as the others. Of the other four with increase in resting heart rate after training, one was felt to be quite anxious on repeat testing in his effort to compete with others in retesting, and another had poor program attendance. The reason for the other two having no decrease in resting heart rate is unknown. Of the nine patients with increase in resting rate after three months of training, five had increase in resting, peak exercise and two-minute postexercise blood pressure, three had a decrease in blood pressure and another had no change. There seems to be, therefore, some common denominator in that greater than half of those with increased resting heart rate after training also had an increase in blood pressure measurements. Interestingly, as seen in Figures 56 through 58, there seems to be a trend to plateau or, in some cases, to increase resting heart rate and systolic blood pressure as well as peak exercise systolic pressure from the three-month to the six-month testing. The reason for this is unknown but could reflect that the best training effect of the program is seen in the first three months. More data involving more patients should be revealing regarding this point. The exercise quotient (Eq) (peak heart rate in beats per minute times peak systolic blood pressure in mm Hg divided by STET in minutes) incorporates more data and seems to have a more consistent trend in evaluating our group of forty-two patients. Although there was no separate group of control subjects, the improved Eq, as represented by decreased magnitude of the Eq number after training, was apparent in all but one of the forty-two patients, and the statistically significant $(p<.01)$ mean value decrease in Eq, both from initial to three-month and from initial to six-month follow-up testing, strongly supports the benefits of the training program. The one patient not improving was one of the three whose resting heart rate increased and was felt to have had an extensive myocardial infarction as manifest by a prolonged period of heart failure while in the hospital with extreme residual electrocardiographic change of infarction.

Few positive correlations can be made regarding body weight and serum studies of cholesterol, triglycerides and uric acid. Of interest is the fact that although forty-one of forty-two patients had decrease in Eq, many had no changes or increase in body weight, in fasting serum cholesterol, triglycerides and uric acid. However, the group of twenty-two patients who had significant decrease in mean value for body weight from initial to follow-up testing at six months, and the group of sixteen patients who had a significant decrease in mean value for triglycerides from initial to six-month follow-up testing, make the data more supportive of a beneficial training effect.

Other factors in our subjects, such as underlying systemic blood pressure abnormalities and dietary indiscretion, may be influential in these results and more data is being gathered on these factors.

Regardless of the lack of uniform individual training effect on blood pressure, heart rate, serum cholesterol, triglycerides and uric acid, the data are suggestive of a beneficial effect on these parameters in the group as a whole. The most vivid and constant effect, however, is seen in the decrease in the Eq which occurred in forty-one of forty-two patients restudied at three months. In conjunction with this, the mean increase in STET in these subjects is significant. However, familiarity with the testing method may cause the latter, more isolated data to be less valid.

The general psychological benefit of the program in all of the subjects who have continued through the three and six-month period is portrayed through statements by the patients that they "feel better." The general "esprit de corps" is obvious, and it is felt that the association of each patient with others who have the same disease problem (i.e. atherosclerotic heart disease) is mutually beneficial for the patients in helping them to accept their disease as its manifestations are explained by their private physicians and the members of the cardiac rehabilitation team.

In conclusion, the aforementioned data suggests that an outpatient gymnasium exercise program for highly selected patients with recent myocardial infarction is feasible and safe. The data suggest that such an exercise program has a beneficial training effect in most patients as manifested by increased STET time and decreased resting and peak exercise systolic blood pressure, resting heart rate, body weight, serum triglycerides and Eq as well as by general psychological improvement.

*Chapter XII*

# RESULTS OF EXERCISE IN

# INDIVIDUAL AND GROUP PROGRAMS

# WITH NONMEDICAL SUPERVISION

### *YMCA "Run for Your Life" Program*

SEVERAL YEARS AGO the authors became interested in the personal and small group exercise of the average middle-aged American male. In accord with this, twenty-three middle-aged male subjects about to begin a Y.M.C.A. "Run for Your Life" jogging program were submitted to a treadmill exercise evaluation prior to and after participating in the three-month jogging program. The schedule followed was Plan "B" of Bowerman and Harris [290] which is an exercise regimen for men in average physical condition. The participants were interviewed by two physicians regarding their occupations, exercise histories and general attitude concerning exercise; they were, in addition, independently cleared by their private physicians for participation in the exercise program.

The subjects had a routine twelve-lead electrocardiogram and maximal treadmill exercise testing as described by Doan *et al.*[194] (The subjects were given a trial run on the treadmill to familiarize them with the procedure before actual testing was begun.) After twelve weeks of organized jogging, re-evaluation was done using the same parameters in order to compare with the pretraining results; the subjects were re-evaluated without being informed as to the results of the initial testing.

Twenty-three male participants were evaluated. The age range was twenty to sixty years with a mean of forty-three years; the weight range was 155 to 213 pounds with a mean of 177 pounds. All subjects were actively employed at the time of their training program. Of the twenty-three participants, fifteen habitually did no more strenuous exercise than golfing; the remainder had engaged in more arduous activity such as sporadic running, swimming and calisthenics.

Of the twenty-three initial electrocardiograms, fourteen were normal; abnormalities seen in the remaining nine were right ventricular conduction defects in four, nonspecific S-T segment changes in three, left axis deviation with an old anterior myocardial infarction in one, and left ventricular hypertrophy in one. Initial maximal treadmill testing revealed frequent premature ventricular contractions in one subject, development of notched P-waves in one, and QRS axis rotation in another. No significant ischemic S-T changes were seen in any of the subjects. The end point symptom was dyspnea in twelve subjects, general fatigue and weakness in one, and leg pain in two. None of the twenty-three participants developed chest pain.

Of the twenty-three subjects, eighteen returned for re-evaluation (some with considerable persuasion); the remainder had either dropped out of the program or were lost to follow-up. One of the eighteen who returned failed to complete the jogging program because of pneumonia; of the other seventeen, seven had missed more than ten of the thirty-five scheduled jogging sessions.

Of the eighteen who had repeat twelve-lead electrocardiograms, one had resolution of S-T segment changes after the training program, one developed a right ventricular conduction defect and one resolved the right ventricular conduction defect. Treadmill evaluation in the group of eighteen revealed no significant electrocardiographic change in sixteen; in one, however, (the same subject with frequent premature ventricular contractions seen prior to training) coupled premature ventricular beats were seen frequently (Fig. 59). In addition, the patient with notched P-waves in the postexercise tracing (before training) had normal P-waves in his post-training treadmill evaluation. Of the eighteen retested, all improved their treadmill endurance by at least one minute; three improved by two minutes, two by three minutes and three by four minutes. The results of this limited evaluation illustrated some of the problems involved in evaluating a physical training program (such as "jogging") and, in addition, point out several advantages as well as potentially dangerous conditions revealed by the treadmill exercise evaluation.

The initial and one of the most difficult problems was that of persuading subjects to return for re-evaluation post-training; this was apparent in that five of the twenty-three subjects (22%) did

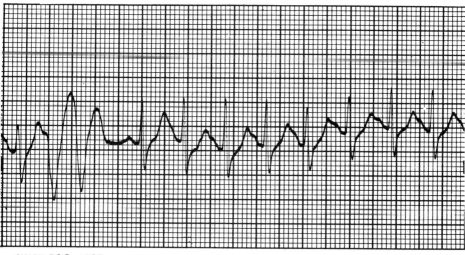

CHART E C G 1000

Figure 59. Electrocardiographic monitor strip showing two consecutive premature ventricular contractions during treadmill testing in subject 2.

not return for retesting. Another significant factor made apparent
was that, of the eighteen returnees, one had dropped out of the
program at the end of fourteen days because of pneumonia and
seven others, for various reasons, had missed more than ten of the
thirty-five training sessions. Therefore, it is obvious that motivation and physical disability play an important role in determining
the success or failure of such a program and its evaluation.

Harris *et al.*[143] evaluated 265 men who completed a twelve-week
jogging program. Beneficial effects included an average decrease in
waist circumference of 1.4 inches, an average drop in systolic and
diastolic pressures of 11.4 mm Hg and 7.8 mm Hg respectively, and
an average weight loss of 7.8 pound in overweight participants.
Adverse effects included seven instances of acute gout and thirty-
four instances of back and leg aches that precipitated withdrawal
from the program.

Stanley and Kezdi [291] studied the cardiopulmonary performance
in thirty-two men before and after a six-month jogging program.
There was no statistically significant improvement as determined
by bicycle ergometer performance and oxygen consumption com-

pared to a matched control group. Motivation varied considerably among the joggers, however, and was felt to be the main reason for lack of significant improvement in fitness.

Regarding the twelve-lead resting electrocardiogram in our group, it is interesting that ten of the twenty-three were abnormal. One twenty-eight-year-old nonathlete had voltage criteria of left ventricular hypertrophy and a forty-four-year-old construction supervisor had changes of an old anterior myocardial infarction although he described no previous cardiovascular symptoms. This latter subject was cleared by his private physician, participated in the program, and improved his treadmill exercise tolerance from eleven to fifteen minutes. It was also of interest that, of the three subjects having nonspecific S-T changes prior to training, two had resolution of these changes in their post-training electrocardiogram.

Although slight to moderate improvement in maximal treadmill endurance was seen in this retested group in the post-training period, the results did not correlate well with adherence to the program, and the test by itself did not seem to reflect fitness derived from the program. It is remarkable that the one subject (with normal resting electrocardiogram) who developed frequent premature ventricular contractions prior to training had coupled premature ventricular contractions so frequently in the post-training evaluations that the physician in charge felt it wise to discontinue the test after seven minutes (prior to the maximal symptomatic end point). No specific changes were noted in the treadmill evaluation of the other subjects, except for one who developed notched P-waves on his initial exercise test.

It is therefore felt that the data obtained from this group of subjects evaluated in pretraining and post-training are inconclusive with regard to change in physical conditioning as measured by the techniques employed (pulse rate and maximal treadmill endurance). However, as Stanley and Kezdi [291] have shown, the duration and intensity of jogging must be controlled if it is to improve cardiopulmonary performance, and improvement in their studies was seen only after four months of intense exercise. Most of the retested subjects in our group, however, stated that they benefited in general and felt better during and after the training program; this is consistent with the results of Mann *et al.*[101] With regard to the subject with electrocardiographic evidence of myocardial infarction and the one with multiple premature ventricular contractions (with coupling), it is apparent that certain cardiac problems or potential problems can be defined with treadmill evaluation and that individuals with such problems may safely complete the training program. For this reason it is felt that preliminary electrocardiographic and treadmill evaluation of subjects beginning exercise programs should be done and subjects should be taught the importance of this evaluation as preventive and therapeutic exercise continues to be popular with coronary-prone American males.

### Exercise in Normal Male Executives

More recently, in order to evaluate a more regimented and better supervised physical activity program, we studied the effects of a six-month organized training program in a group of healthy white male sedentary executives.[292] Predominantly sedentary white male executives employed by a private life insurance firm in Atlanta, Georgia, were studied before and after six months of participation in an established, organized physical training program. The program was available to the executives in their home office building, and some tenants in other businesses were also included. There were facilities and equipment for weight lifting and isometric exercise (Fig. 60) as well as nonmotorized treadmills, handball and paddleball courts (Fig. 61) and a roof jogging track (Fig. 62). Organized exercise classes were held regularly during the office hours and ample time was provided for physical training during the day as desired by the participants. Most participants exercised three or four times weekly for periods of forty-five to sixty minutes.

Exercise testing was performed in the Georgia Baptist Hospital exercise laboratory. The participants were tested only once prior to their participation in the training program. The maximal treadmill exercise test, as described by Doan and Bruce,[194] was utilized with a motor-driven, variable grade, multispeed treadmill. Cardiopulmonary resuscitation equipment was available, and both a physician and registered nurse were present during testing.

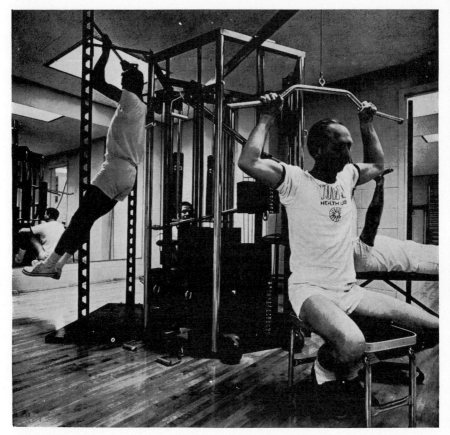

Figure 60. View of exercise utilizing a Universal machine.

Initially, a brief cardiac history and brief physical examination, as well as a resting supine, pre-exercise twelve-lead electrocardiogram (ECG) were performed. If any of these or the subsequent exercise test revealed an abnormality, further examination by the insurance company's internist, or perferably a cardiologist, was recommended to the company's physical training director. If the subject recovered normally (heart rate returning to the 120 beats per minute level or less in three minutes) [284] the test was terminated. If there was delayed recovery of the pulse, an abnormal blood pressure response, rhythm disturbance or sustained S-T segment abnormality, rhythm strip recordings were continued until such a time

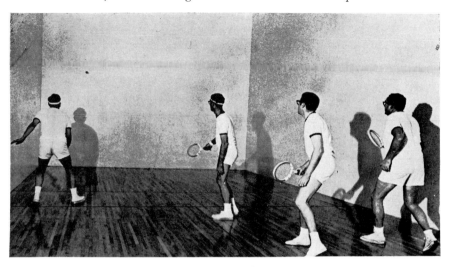

Figure 61. Views of paddleball court with executives actively engaged in game.

(individualized for each subject) deemed sufficient for safe termination of the postexercise evaluation. After testing, the subject was told of his performance and was encouraged to return for repeat exercise testing after approximately six months of his participation in the active exercise program.

The heart rate-systolic blood pressure product (RPP) was calculated as an index of myocardial oxygen consumption ($MVO_2$). Each subject was evaluated regarding his overall participation in the exercise program, (i.e. his regularity of participation, the estimated number of calories expanded during each session, the improvement in his performance of activities, his willingness to participate in the studies and his maximal treadmill exercise test [MTT] performance).

Although fifty subjects were initially tested, only 60 percent (thirty of fifty) were restudied. The mean age for the subjects restudied was 42.7 years (range twenty-eight to sixty-five years).

During the six months of training, there were many cancellations of the treadmill exercise test. Conflicts in schedules, minor illnesses and intermittent periods of poor exercise program participation accounted for cancellations and prevented retesting for

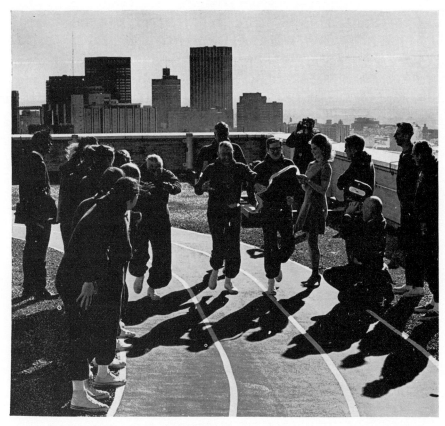

Figure 62. View of roof track (sixteenth of a mile in circumference). Subjects are assisting in a television news story. The Atlanta skyline is seen in the background.

some subjects. The problems included busy work schedules, company transfers to distant cities, musculoskeletal injuries as a direct result of exercising (including a ruptured Achilles tendon and a fractured carpal bone) and a positive test for ischemic heart disease (the private physician preferred no retesting).

The symptoms most frequently noted on MTT in the retested group of thirty subjects were leg fatigue, general fatigue and shortness of breath. Arrhythmias and conduction abnormalities occurred during MTT in 15 percent (nine of sixty) of the tests. Included were premature atrial beats (1), premature nodal beats

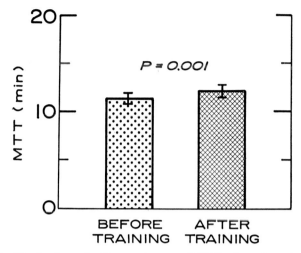

Figure 63. Maximal treadmill exercise test (MTT) times in minutes before and after the training period. See text for discussion.

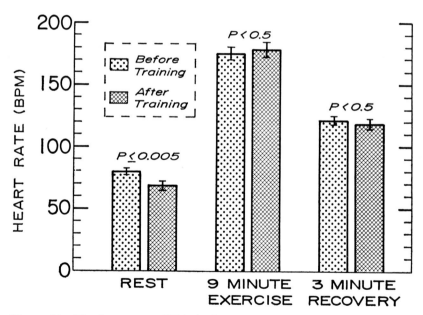

Figure 64. The heart rate (HR) in beats per minute (BPM) for the resting, nine-minute exercising and three-minute recovery periods (p values are noted). See text for discussion.

(1), first degree atrioventricular (A-V) block (twice in one subject), premature ventricular beats (PVB) (four in three subjects) and supraventricular tachycardia (1). All arrhythmias resolved with training except two subjects with PVB's and the one with A-V block. For the thirty subjects restudied, the average (MTT) time of 12.9 minutes before training increased to 14.3 minutes after the training period (See Fig. 63) (p < 0.001). The corresponding resting heart rate (supine) significantly decreased from an initial average of 79.4 beats per minute (BPM) to 67.7 BPM on retesting (p < .05). The three-minute recovery rate BPM (sitting) decreased on initial testing from an average of 121.3 BPM to 119.9 BPM after training (p < 0.5) (Fig. 64). The heart rate and blood pressure used in the data during exercise were those recorded at the end of nine minutes duration on the treadmill (end of stage 3) for all participants.

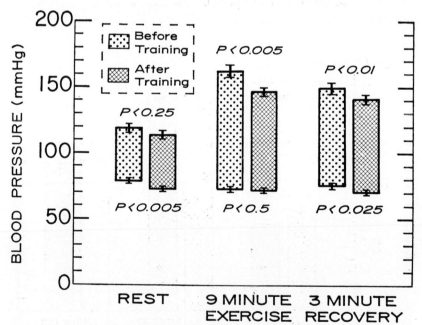

Figure 65. The blood pressure (BP) in mmHg (systolic above each bar and diastolic below) in the resting, nine-minute exercising and three-minute recovery periods before and after training. Means and standard deviations are displayed within bars for the corresponding BP (p values are noted). See text for discussion.

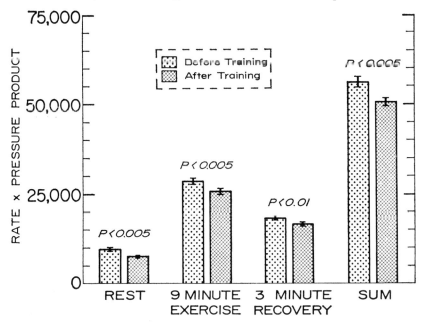

Figure 66. The mean rate-pressure products are shown before and after training for the resting, nine-minute exercising, and three-minute recovery periods. The sum of these three periods before and after training is also displayed. P values and T-test values are noted for each set of paired numbers. Means and standard deviations are recorded within each bar.

The resting blood pressure (BP) decreased from an initial average 118/78 mm Hg to 113/72 mm Hg on retesting (p < 0.25). The blood pressure after nine minutes of exercise decreased significantly (p < 0.005) from an average control level of 172/73 mm Hg to 146/71 mm Hg on retesting. The three-minute recovery BP decreased from an initial average of 149/75 mm Hg to 141/70 mm Hg on retesting (p < 0.025) (Fig. 65).

The systolic blood pressure (SBP) of the subjects sitting after three minutes of recovery was 15 mm Hg or more higher than the SBP after nine minutes of exercise in twenty-one (70%) of the thirty subjects. In these twenty-one subjects the average increase of the recovery SBP above the nine-minute exercising level was 34.9 mm Hg (range 18 to 70 mm Hg). In seven of the twenty-one subjects, the SBP during recovery rest periods was equal to or greater than 200 mm Hg with an average elevation of 35.7 mm Hg (range 10 to 79 mm Hg).

The mean values of the RPP's for the thirty participants decreased from control values for the resting, the nine-minute exercise and the three-minute postexercise recovery period as seen in Figure 66. The sum of these RPP's for each of the retested participants decreased significantly (p < 0.005) in 76.6 percent (twenty-three of thirty) of the subjects.

In the present study a group of thirty normal, predominately sedentary male executives were studied before and after a six-month physical training period in a supervised program. In this group there were difficulties in maintaining the subjects in continuous participation in the program and in scheduling the subjects for treadmill retesting. A major problem with this study was the lack of reliability due to the absence of multiple testings in the pre- and post-training periods. This was produced, in part, because of the work status of the subjects tested. The group consisted of executive businessmen who were aggressive, independent and demanding of others and of themselves. These reasons may have accounted for their decreased motivation and enthusiasm for participation, and also their participation in both the training program and the exercise testing after the initial novelty of the training program waned.

There were difficulties in scheduling because of prearranged and fixed periods during the week for treadmill retesting. These times were inconvenient for some of the subjects whose own schedules produced conflicts. During the winter season, minor illnesses and days of "not feeling their best" caused a number of subjects to reschedule the treadmill retest. Weekends and holiday festivities and periods of associated minimal physical activities resulted in problems associated with feelings of less than peak physical fitness, lack of enthusiasm for retesting and, therefore, many cancellations and rescheduled treadmill retests resulted. Minor orthopedic complications such as various "strains and sprains" of ligaments and muscles were associated with the exercise training. These and other previous orthopedic surgical procedures in a few subjects prevented their optimal performance on initial and follow-up testings. Of interest is the fact that there seemed to be some correla-

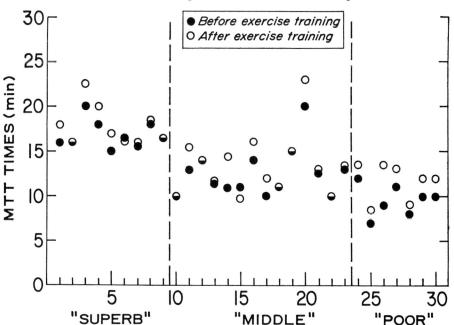

Figure 67. Data showing correlation between control MTT and degree of subsequent participation of the subjects in the program. See text.

tion between an individuals' control MTT and the degree of subsequent participation in the program (Fig. 67).

Comparison of the pre- and post-training data shown in Figures 63 through 66 reveals several pertinent points. The recovery HR's on retesting did not significantly decrease. This abnormal recovery may reflect irregular and inconsistent exercise training on the part of the participants. Blood pressure (BP) measurements with reliable accuracy beyond stage 4 (nine minutes) of the maximal treadmill test were technically inconsistent. These inconsistencies resulted because of difficulties in recording the BP with the excessive arm motion and the variations in BP produced by gripping the side rails. Therefore, a technically stable and constantly reliable BP measurement was common to all subjects: the nine-minute recording (at the end of stage 3). Frequently, the systolic (S) BP was observed to increase early in the recovery period (including the measurement taken immediately after exercise testing and in the first and second minutes of the recovery period) above that recorded at the nine-minute point in the maximal treadmill test. This "recovery rebound" has been noted in walking MTT's by Fraser and Chapman [293] and Logan and Bruce; [294] however, "exertional hypotension," as they described did not occur.

Hiss and Lamb [295] have tabulated the occurrence of various arrhythmias recorded at rest in apparently healthy male air force cadet applicants. The incidence of premature ventricular beats (PVBs) increased with increasing age. Lamb and Hiss [295] also studied the influence of exercise stress upon the incidence of PVBs. It was their opinion that PVBs occurring during and/or after exertion were innocuous unless accompanied by clinical evidence supporting the presence of underlying heart disease. The epidemiologic study from Tecumseh, Michigan,[166] however, correlated the occurrence of antecedent PVBs at rest with an increased incidence of manifest coronary atherosclerotic heart disease and sudden death during the subsequent years. The prevalence of PVBs also increased with age and occurred more frequently in men than women. In our study, there were no premature beats at rest and the arrhythmias that did occur with exercise were not consistently associated with either positive family histories for coronary atherosclerotic heart disease or increased age.

In spite of difficulties in evaluating the exercise training in this group, the average maximal treadmill exercise times, resting heart rates, blood pressures and rate-pressure products, as specific parameters of cardiac function, improved after the training period.

In the evaluation of our data, the "recovery rebound" (a hypertensive response as measured by either a rise in SBP of 15 mm Hg above the exercising SBP or a systolic elevation of 200 mm Hg during the recovery resting-sitting period) was frequent. The relationship of this response to inadequate training and/or to a variation of latent or labile blood pressure is unknown.

Regular and consistent exercise through organized physical training programs for six months may produce beneficial effects as manifest by increased post-training MTT and decreased BP, resting HR and RPP; these beneficial effects are supported by other data.[297-300,22] In the present study, it was not possible to state whether the apparent improvement was due to the exercise training or to other factors such as familiarity with the method, decreased anxiety or increased motivation and greater effort. Subjects who had higher exercise testing scores were more likely to attend physical training programs than subjects with lower scores. If the apparent improvement in performance during exercise testing can be proven to lower subsequent morbidity or mortality from coronary atherosclerotic heart disease, then more diligent efforts to increase the number of organized physical training programs at adequately equipped facilities at all socioeconomic levels should be encouraged, and the need for exercise testing should be emphasized.

### Summary

The results of studies in these two different groups of somewhat independent exercises are supportive of the benefits of exercise both with regard to "general feeling" and objective data (in the second group). The lack of significant cardiac complications with the training makes such activity feasible and safe; the safety, however, is thought to be contingent on proper exercise testing.

The problem with follow-up testing and persistent attendance in this type of program, as compared to that of the program described in Chapter XI, are apparent. It is felt, however, that the advantages outweigh the disadvantages and such activities should be encouraged.

*Chapter XIII*

# CARDIAC REHABILITATION
# IN OTHER COUNTRIES

T HE PURPOSE OF this section is to review briefly the activities and results of several programs of exercise training for patients with coronary heart disease that are presently underway in other countries. These programs are located in Helsinki (Finland), Goteberg (Sweden) and Hohenried (Germany). One of the authors (GFF) recently visited each of these programs and personally interviewed the physician directors and observed the exercise testing and training activities. This discussion will include current data (much of which is unpublished) derived from these programs, and the figures will include photographs of testing and training activities.

It is felt that international interest in physical training is increasing and that the experiences of other countries have in the past, and will in the future, have considerable impact on our attitude toward exercise in the management of coronary heart disease. It is obvious that each population differs in baseline physical activities and in physical activity after myocardial infarction; also the coronary risk factors (such as hypertension, smoking and lipid abnormalities) vary from one country to another. Hopefully, this section will not only inform the reader but also elicit critique regarding methods of testing and training utilized in these countries compared to those described in American programs.

### Helsinki, Finland

Kentala,[148] in the second Department of Medicine at Helsinki University, has recently summarized the results of exercise training in 298 consecutive male patients under sixty-five years who were treated in the hospital with a diagnosis of acute myocardial infarction. The patients were divided in the hospital into a control group and a training group by their year of birth in order to make a controlled study in physical rehabilitation after myocardial infarction. Forty-five patients died in the hospital. Patients with other severe diseases were excluded from the follow-up study. Of the patients discharged from the hospital, 158 met the diagnostic criteria of acute myocardial infarction defined in this study, and lived so close to the hospital that they could be accepted for a twelve-month follow-up study of supervised physical training. Seventy-seven with a mean age of fifty-three years made up the training group. The physical working capacity of these men was measured by means of a bicycle ergometer test six to eight weeks after the infarction.

After this test the members of the training group were given an opportunity to participate in supervised training exercises at first twice, and later, three times a week. In these exercises the patient's heart rate was kept for twenty minutes about ten beats below the level reached at the first maximal test. The loads were increased when the working heart rate slowed. In order to ensure uniform basic treatment, all the patients in both the control group and the training group attended the outpatient department once a month for consultation with the author. In addition to the first exercise test, the patients underwent maximal exercise tests five and twelve months after the infarction. Clinical findings, anthropometric measurements, ECG, chest x-rays, serum lipid values and the two-hour glucose tolerance test were recorded at these times.

There were only minor differences between the groups in the anamnestic data, anthropometric measurements and clinical findings recorded in the hospital. A statistically significant difference was observed in the serum cholesterol value three weeks after the infarction; it was 238 mg/100 ml in the control and 256 mg/100 ml in the training group (p < 0.05). The vital capacity (in percent of the predicted value) was one hundred in the control and ninety-five in the training group (p < 0.05).

Physical working capacity at the first measurement six to eight weeks after the infarction was 498 kpm/minute in the control and 470 kpm/minute in the training group (Fig. 68). The corresponding mean heart rates at maximal load were 129 and 128 beats/minute.

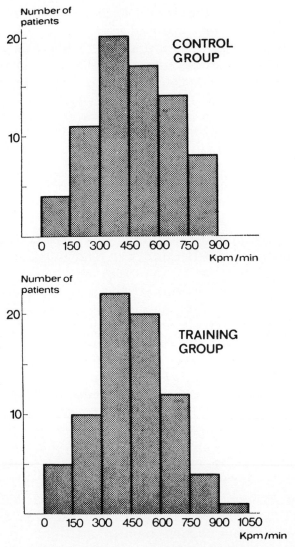

Figure 68. Bar graph showing the distribution of physical work capacity six to eight weeks after myocardial infarction in the control group and in the training group (Courtesy of Kentala).

The initial physical working capacity was only approximately half of that of healthy men of the same age and occupation. The variation in physical working capacity was wide, ranging from under 150 kpm/minute to 1,050 kpm/minute

Stepwise regression analysis was applied to find out the determinants of physical working capacity six to eight weeks after the infarction. Variables of the first myocardial infarction recorded during the hospital phase turned out to be of relatively small significance except variables related to cardiac failure. The patient's physical fitness prior to the infarction had an important influence on the subsequent physical working capacity.

The feasibility of participation in the regular examinations was good, i.e. almost all the patients attended. However, it was possible to implement an adequate, supervised physical training program for only a minority of the training group. Four patients died within five months of the infarction. Poor functional capacity precluded participation in the training program for a further twelve of the seventy-seven patients in the training group. Of the remaining sixty-one patients, twenty-nine participated adequately up to the first follow-up study five months after the infarction. Later, the number of patients with an adequate attendance rate diminished further to only ten between the sixth and twelfth months. However, in addition to these patients, another sixteen patients maintained physical activity of training level on their own accord.

The physical activity of the control group also increased. After a year, eleven control patients maintained physical activity of full training level.

This shows that physical reconditioning can be carried out completely on the patient's own initiative. To sum up, supervised physical training appeared to be indicated and feasible in only about one-fifth of an unselected infarction series. Especially patients with poor prognostic features need close supervision of the physical training, if this is applied.

One recurrence of infarction occurred during the training sessions. There was no difference between the control and training groups in morbidity and mortality (Figure 69 a&b). Locomotor complications were few.

Because the intergroup difference in physical activity turned

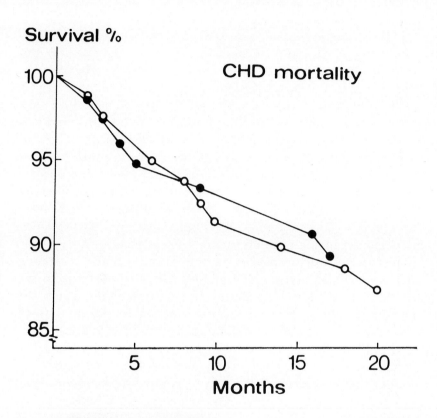

Figure 69a. Graph showing survival rates during the twenty-month follow-up period in the control and training group (Courtesy of Kentala).

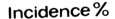

Incidence%

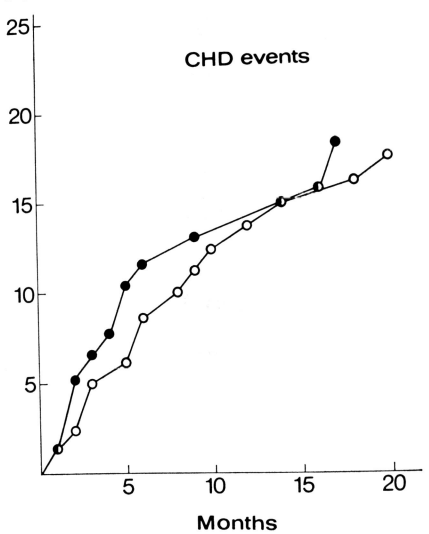

o Control group

● Training group

Figure 69b. Graph showing the incidence of coronary heart disease (CHD) events during the follow-up period in the control and training group (Courtesy of Kentala).

out to be small for the reasons mentioned above, it follows that no statistically significant difference in physical working capacity was established in the follow-up study between the original control and training groups. Both groups displayed a clear decrease in the heart rate-blood pressure product measured at the same submaximal load, while an increase was elicited at maximal work load.

Those individuals in whom supervised physical training was feasible, i.e. with an attendance rate of 70 percent or more, improved their physical working capacity markedly more (p < 0.0025) than the other members of the training group by the five-month test, although the mean initial capacities were practically the same.

On the basis of an interview made at the twelve-month follow-up the whole patient series was regrouped into those with a training level physical activity and those without, regardless of whether they were initially in the control or training groups. The physical working capacity of the high activity subgroup increased significantly more than that of the others by the five-month follow-up examination (p < 0.0001), and started from better initial capacity (p < 0.05). This increase in the course of one year was 56 percent in the patients maintaining the high level of physical activity (Grade III), against 26 percent for the rest of the total series divided in this way.

The initial physical working capacity six to eight weeks after the infarction was the most important single variable in the training group predicting the physical working capacity achieved by training in twelve months. Next in the stepwise regression analysis came the average training heart rate, participation rate, FEV 1.0, cardiac failure complicating the acute infarction, paradoxical cardiac pulsation and heart volume.

The subjects participating adequately in supervised physical training showed the most distinct decrease in the skin fold measurements and weight loss. These patients were also somewhat better able to give up smoking. Further, the patients with training level activity gave initially significantly (p < 0.001) more numerous Q-QS findings in accordance with Minnesota Code, but they disappeared considerably faster in the course of the twelve-month follow-up. No corresponding changes were noted in regard to ST-T alterations.

Return to work was not influenced by the supervised physical training. Sixty-eight percent of the patients in the total series who had been at work before the current infarction and who were alive twelve months after it returned to work. This percentage is only 26.5 in an unselected series from the Ischemic Heart Disease Register of Helsinki. It became evident that just regular follow-up examinations by a doctor, measurement of physical working capacity, adequate medical therapy and the sense of security given by continuous contact with a physician contribute at least as much to return to work as does supervised physical training. The number of sustained myocardial infarctions was the most important determinant of retirement in the multiple discriminating analysis. The patients who retired in conjunction with the current infarction were distinguished from the rest of the series in that they had been in the physically heaviest work; these jobs had been frequently too heavy for their actual work capacity. The myocardial infarction appeared to be overestimated in the evaluation of the working capacity of the patient, leading fairly readily to his retirement on pension. At other times a patient with ischemic heart disease may have to work for a long time in conditions that are beyond his functional capacity without vacation or pension even being considered.

The prognosis for the next one to two postinfarction years was most clearly associated with paradoxical cardiac pulsation noted during the treatment of acute infarction. If this finding was easily established on palpation of the chest, it implied a poor prognosis. Other predictors of poor prognosis were an increasing frequency of ventricular extrasystoles during the hospital stay, low arterial blood pressure, poor physical working capacity measured six to eight weeks after the infarction, and various signs of cardiac or respiratory failure. Whether the patient belonged to the control or training group was of no prognostic importance.

On the basis of the study by Kentala some physicians in Helsinki now feel less enthusiastic about the benefits of programs of supervised physical activities for patients with recent myocardial infarction. They, however, feel that this could reflect the characteristics of their specific population sample and do not attempt to apply this rigidly to other populations.

The noted differences in skin fold measurements, weight loss and ease of giving up cigarette smoking in the supervised trained group as opposed to the control group is certainly encouraging as regards alleviation of coronary risk factors. This may influence the future, especially in lieu of the high intake of saturated fats in the Finnish population—i.e. cheeses and milk, the latter reportedly in the range of one liter per person per day.

### Goteborg, Sweden

At Sahlgrens Hospital, University of Goteborg, an outpatient facility has been utilized for exercising patients with recent myocardial infarction. The facility is part of the physical therapy department and the exercise program is under the supervision of the physiotherapists. The program consists of sessions of walking and calisthenics three times weekly. Personal conversation with Dr. Lars Wilhelmsen reveals that the physician staff has been pleased with their results in programmed exercise in patients with recent myocardial infarction. They feel that one of the most important aspects of this type of patient management has been the evolution of methods of patient and family education and the study of coronary risk factors.

One of the studies reported relating to the experience in Goteberg was with primary intervention of high risk factors related to myocardial infarction. In this, Wilhelmsen *et al.*[301] described a preventive trial aiming at treatment of the risk factors—hypertension, elevated serum cholesterol, smoking and, to some degree, low physical activity. At the time of the study report, 305 subjects had been found with previously undiagnosed and untreated hypertension. Of these, 210 have been placed on drug therapy and, in most, blood pressure has become normal. Regarding hypercholesterolemia, diet information is provided by a doctor and a dietician. Clofibrate and nicotinic acid are also utilized accordingly to the type of lipid abnormality. A seasonal variation has been noted with the mean serum cholesterol recorded of 233 mgm% in December and 256 mgm% in March.

With regard to smoking, of special interest has been the utilization of an antismoking clinic for those who smoked less than fifteen cigarettes per day. The introduction information meeting comprised around forty participants followed by group sessions of seven to ten participants. Only rarely were they treated individually. All smokers received information about the positive consequences of not smoking and were advised on steps in a cessation program, although they were advised to stop completely. Some decreased their tobacco consumption by changing from cigarettes to cigars or pipes.

In addition, chewing gum containing nicotine has been used in the early cessation period. Of the 295 men who have entered the program, ninety-three (32%) have stopped smoking completely and sixty-five (22%) have reduced their smoking by less than 50 percent.

Little emphasis was placed on physical activity except for increasing activity in those with very low levels of activity. The specifics are not described.

Later in the same year Gustafson *et al.*[302] reported a series of 229 postmyocardial infarction patients studied up to two years following hospitalization with comparison to a random population sample of men of comparable age. Hyperlipoproteinemia, cholesterol and triglycerides elevation were more common in myocardial infarction patients, especially in the younger group. There was a trend toward higher mortality among patients with hyperlipoproteinemia. Types II A and B were very common in young patients. Serum cholesterol values were significantly higher in the youngest patients and serum triglyceride higher in the controls in age groups forty < forty-six to fifty and fifty-one to fifty-five years.

More recently unpublished data by Wilhelmsen and Tibblin [303] (obtained by personal interviews) has been revealing regarding coronary risk factors. Nine hundred seventy-three men (all age fifty) were recruited from a general Swedish urban population. Of the 855 participants, 834 were coronary heart disease free on entry and have been observed for nine years and four months. All except two of fifty-five deaths were autopsied. Twenty-five near-fatal and nineteen fatal cases of coronary heart disease occurred.

By a multiple model, nine probable risk factors were analyzed.

Serum cholesterol, smoking, systolic blood pressure, dyspnea and conviction for drunkenness were significantly related to coronary heart disease, but not serum triglycerides, hematocrit or social mobility (place of birth), while physical inactivity during work showed a slight tendency to relationship.

The predictive capability of the logistic function (with cholesterol, smoking and systolic blood pressure) was tested in another randomly selected population sample of 5,146 men (ages fifty-one to fifty-five years) and found to be quite accurate. Thus, it was possible to isolate the highest decile group of men with a twenty-nine times higher risk of suffering coronary heart disease than the lowest decile.

Thus, efforts in Sweden (particularly in Goteberg) seem to be predominantly directed toward risk factor detection and modification. The structure of the city registry in Goteborg and the accessability of data and cooperation of the registry with the physician investigators make such studies most realistic and rewarding. The studies being done at the time under the direction of Dr. Wilhelmsen are most impressive, and the methodology seems worthy of the stature of an international model for coronary risk factor detection, evaluation and modification.

### Hohenried, Germany

By far the most elaborate and extensive cardiac exercise rehabilitation center in Europe (seen by the author) was that at Klinik, Hohenreid, Germany, twenty kilometers south of Munich on the Starnberger Sea. The facility (seen in aerial view in Fig. 70) has approximately 600 beds with a four-bed coronary care unit; the total surrounding area encompasses almost twenty acres. The area was originally the land surrounding a large castle (seen in Fig. 71 as it relates to the rehabilitation center); the castle is now used as a recreation facility for the physicians and staff of the rehabilitation center. The center is a modern unit complex with a connecting closed corrider. There is a large gymnasium (Fig. 72) and an indoor pool with additional area for a sauna and various types of physical therapy. In the adjacent outdoor area there is minigolf (Fig. 73) and lawn bowling (Fig. 74). The beach and sea nearby are utilized as a part of the daily recreational and training activities (Fig. 75).

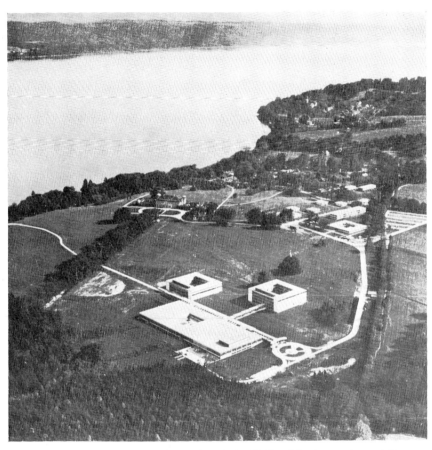

Figure 70. Aerial view of the Hohenried Klinik with the castle and Starnberger Sea in the background.

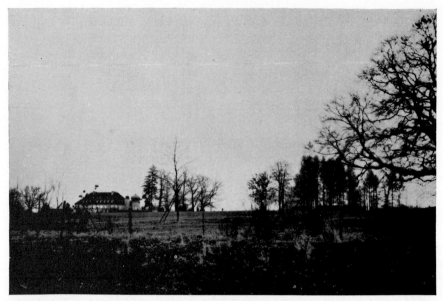

Figure 71.  Castle about which Hohenried Klinik is built.

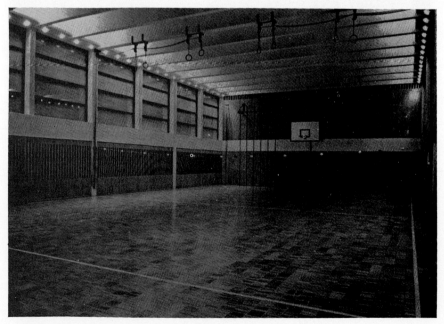

Figure 72.  View of gymnasium facility at Hohenried Klinik.

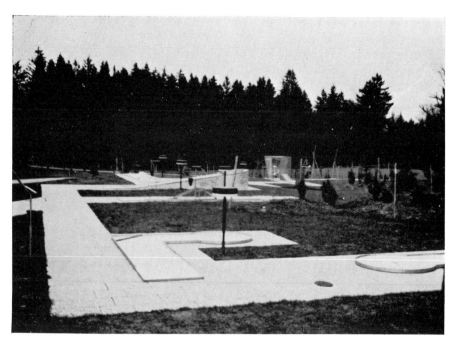

Figure 73. View of the minigolf course at Hohenried Klinik.

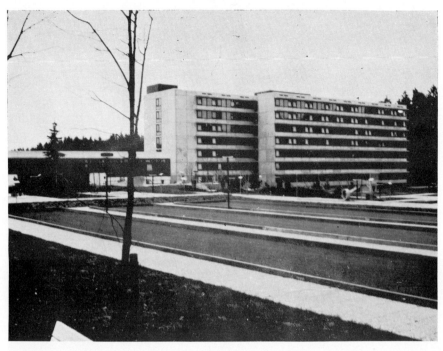

Figure 74. View of the lawn bowling lanes with Klinik buildings in background.

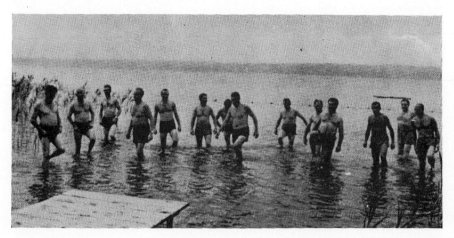

Figure 75. Bathers seen in shallow water of the sea in daily beach activities.

The patient population is obtained by private referral—mainly from the southern part of Germany. The population is of middle class derivation and the rehabilitation program is supported by national health insurance. Referral of patients takes place from four to six months after myocardial infarction and at any one time there are approximately 550 patients in the facility. Each patient remains at the Klinik for a period of six weeks in his own private room (Fig. 76) and is allowed visits by his family only on weekends. After initial bicycle ergometer stress testing (Fig. 77) the patient undergoes a progressive program of training and recreation. The activities include running, calisthenics (Fig. 78), minigolf, lawn bowling and swimming (Fig. 79). In addition to the above, the patients are trained by bicycle ergometry twice weekly at which time they have constant telemetry monitoring of their electrocardiogram (Fig. 80). After the six-week period the patients are discharged and followed by consultation in the rehabilitation clinic and in their own homes.

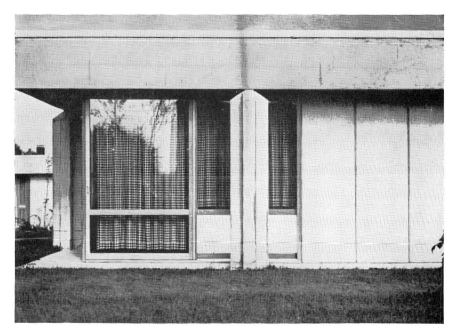

Figure 76. Outside view of individual living units.

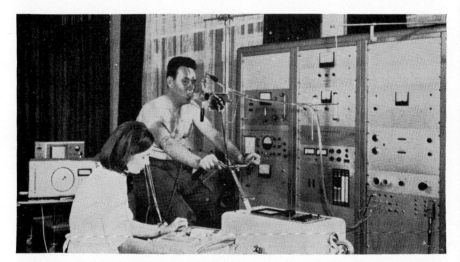

Figure 77. Photo of patient undergoing ergometry stress testing prior to exercise training at Hohenried Klinik.

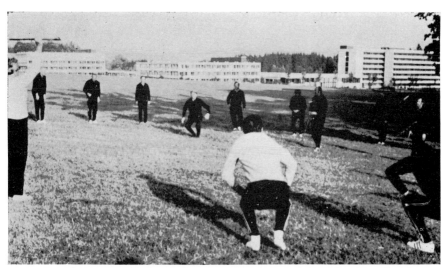

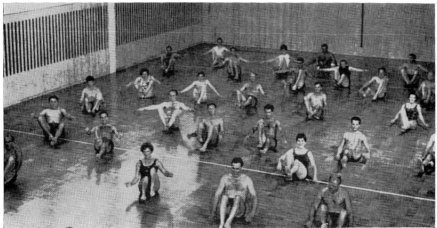

Figure 78. Views of calisthenics—both outside (a) and inside the gymnasium (b).

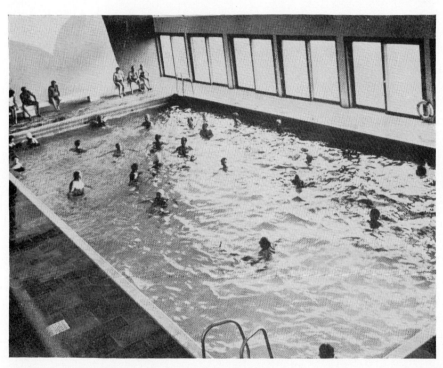

Figure 79.  Patients in gym pool during daily swimming activities.

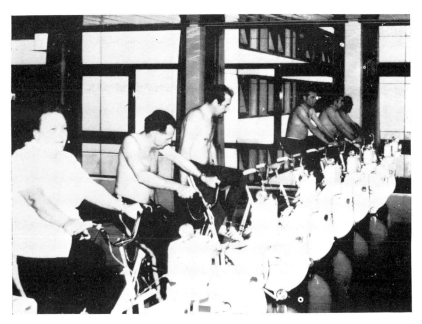

Figure 80. Patients having follow-up exercise testing during telemetry ECG monitoring.

In addition to the 550 postmyocardial infarction patients, the Klinik usually has seventy-five to one hundred coronary-prone patients in training. These patients spend four weeks at the Klinik and have a similar program to the postmyocardial infarction patients; however, it is more strenuous and involves more use of isometric maneuvers such as weight lifting.

In 1972 Stocksmeier and Halhuber [304] reported preliminary results of the Hohenried longitudinal cross section study of patients with myocardial infarction. Patients under comprehensive care for myocardial infarction were observed for ten years and information concerning recurrence of myocardial infarction and mortality, readjustment of mode of living, capacity to earn and living and diet utilization ratio were recorded and evaluated. In ninety-two workers and salaried employees suffering from myocardial infarction, an adjustment of diet lasting eleven months could be achieved by intensive consultation in the rehabilitation clinic and in the household, which showed a change in the ratio of polyunsaturated to saturated fatty acid of 0.3 to 1.2. During the six weeks in rehabilitation it was possible to reduce significantly the mean levels of body weight, blood pressure and blood lipids of 273 myocardial infarction patients. The effect of the modification lasted at least nine months after discharge from the rehabilitation center. As about one-third of the 490 myocardial infarction patients accepted in the meantime received follow-up treatment (early rehabilitation), the time between the occurrence of the myocardial infarction and return to work was of interest. It was found that with the follow-up treatment there was an advance of about three months in beginning work. It was felt, however, that the only way to obtain sufficient information as to whether such an advance is beneficial or harmful to the patient is by prolonging the duration of the study.

In summary, the Klinik Hohenried is the epitomy of an all-encompassing facility for cardiac rehabilitation. The thirty-five physicians and fifty nurses along with physiotherapists and other personnel who supervised the program form an adequate number of capable staff. The experience in evaluation of patient data is inconclusive at this point, but suggests a benefit of more rapid return to work and a consistent fall in blood pressure and blood lipids up to a year thereafter. As with other programs, there is a need for a longer duration of study involving more patients before conclusive evidence can be available.

# Chapter XIV

# SUMMARY

IN THIS BOOK we have attempted to update, review and discuss the somewhat controversial issue of exercise and coronary heart disease and have covered historical aspects as well as a discussion of the advantages and disadvantages. It is felt that the use of exercise in the proper manner will utilize the advantages and tend to eliminate the disadvantages, complications and risks. In dealing with exercise we feel that it can be made proper by recommending the use of those types of physical activity that affect and increase the work (myocardial oxygen consumption) of the heart, thus tending to condition (train) the patient to the point at which he can obtain higher levels of physical activity without increasing the work of the heart.

We have also emphasized the value of exercise testing of patients to determine the heart rate and blood pressure response to certain levels of exercise in order to recommend the safest and best level of exercise for their physical conditioning; in addition, we recommend this for detection of arrhythmias and ischemic S-T segment changes and the patient's subjective response to exercise.

Lastly, we have commented on the issue of proper exercise in the alteration of risk factors; additional well-controlled studies are needed. This is particularly true in view of the International Cooperative Study on Cardiovascular Epidemiology, which did not show a clear association between coronary proneness and physical inactivity.[91] In an editorial comment on the latter results, Paul correctly states that "this is surely a complex issue, and from this kind of evidence the value of physical exercise in coronary disease prevention should neither be readily dismissed nor be adopted with evangelistic fervor as some have." [11,305] We favor a common sense approach to exercise prescription, recognizing that controlled studies are nonexistent in this area.

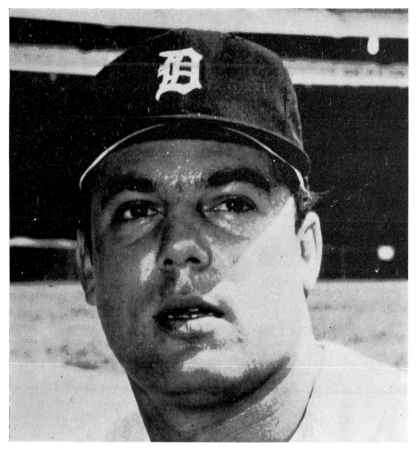

Figure 81. Major league baseball pitcher who returned to stardom following a myocardial infarction. (Photo courtesy of Ed Thilenius TV-5, Atlanta, and the Detroit Tiger baseball club).

Cardiac rehabilitation has many faces, ranging from the motivation of an executive to reduce coronary risk factors to the return of a professional baseball player to active status following a myocardial infarction (Fig. 81). As an important part of the rehabilitation process, exercise is inexpensive, enjoyable to most and so far appears safe for the coronary-prone individual and for the postcoronary patient if done properly. The latter necessitates thorough preliminary evaluation and medical supervision. If the only beneficial effect of exercise in the coronary patient was an *alleviation of fear, anxiety and sense of impending doom,* that alone would validate the time and cost of research in this area to date.

# REFERENCES

*Chapter I*

1. Enos, W.F., Holmes, R.H., and Beyer, J.: Coronary disease among United States soldiers killed in action in Korea. *JAMA, 152:*1090–1093, 1953.
2. Mason, J.K.: Asymptomatic disease of coronary arteries in young men. *Br Med J, 2:*1234–1237, 1963.
3. Viel, B., Donoso, S., and Salcedo, D.: Coronary atherosclerosis in persons dying violently. *Arch Intern Med, 122:*97–103, 1968.
4. *An Old Age, X34* (James Logan-translator). Cited in *Familiar Medical Quotations* (Strauss M. Ed., Boston, Little, Brown) 169, 1968.
5. Fox, S.M. III, and Skinner, J.S.: Physical activity and cardiovascular health. *Am J Cardiol, 14:*731–746, 1964.
6. Parmley, L.F.: Proceedings of the National Conference on Exercise in the prevention, in the evaluation, in the treatment of heart disease. *J SC Med Assoc, 65:*i, 1969.
7. *The Spectator,* Vol II, No. 115 (July 12, 1911). Cited in ref. 4, p. 165.
8. Adams, C.W.: Symposium on exercise and the heart (Introduction). *Am J Cardiol, 30:*713–715, 1972.
9. Easton, J.: *Human longevity,* London, Salisburg 1799, p. xi, xxvi.
10. Alexander, J.K.: Exercise and coronary heart disease. *Cardiovasc Res Cent Bull, 8:*2–7, 1969.
11. White, Paul Dudley: (Personal Communication), 1969.
12. Currens, J.H., and White, P.D.: Half a century of running: Clinical, physiological and autopsy findings in the case of Clarence DeMar, ("Mr. Marathon"). *N Engl J Med, 265:*988–993, 1961.
13. Chapman, C.B.: Edward Smith (1818–1874) Physiologist, human ecologist, reformer. *J Hist Med, 22:*1–26, 1967.
14. Smith, E.: Inquiries into the quantity of air inspired throughout the day and night, and under the influence of exercise, food, medicine and temperature. *Proc Roy Soc, 8:*451–456, 1857.
15. Smith, E.: Report on the sanitary circumstances of tailors in London. In 6th Ed. Rep Med Officer Primary Council with Appendix, 1863. London, H.M. Stationary Office 416–430, 1864.

*Chapter II*

16. Fletcher, G.F.: Exercise and the heart. *ACCESS, 2:* No. 5, 1970.
17. Falls, H.B.: Proceedings of the national conference on exercise in the prevention, in the evaluation and in the treatment of heart disease. The relative energy requirements of various physical activities in relation to physiological strain. *J SC Med Assoc, 65:*8, 1969.

18. Wells, J.G., Balke, B., and Van Fossan, D.D.: Lactic acid accumulation during work; a suggested standardization of work classification. *J Appl Physiol, 10:*51–55, 1957.

19. Sarnoff, S.J., Braunwald, F., and Welch, G.F., Jr., *et al.:* Hemodynamic determinants of oxygen consumption of the heart with special reference to the tension time index. *Am J Physiol, 192:*148–156, 1958.

20. Monroe, R.G., and Frence, G.N.: Left ventricular pressure-volume relationships and myocardial oxygen consumption in the isolated heart. *Circ Res, 9:*362–374, 1961.

21. Robinson, B.F.: Relation of heart rate and systolic blood pressure to the onset of pain in angina pectoris. *Circulation, 35:*1073–1083, 1967.

22. Mitchell, J.H., Sproule, B.J., and Chapman, C.B.: The physiological meaning of the maximal oxygen intake test. *J Clin Invest, 37:*538–547, 1958.

23. Frick, M.H., Konttinen, A., and Sarajas, H.S.: Effects of physical training on circulation at rest and during exercise. *Am J Cardiol, 12:*142–147, 1963.

24. Saltin, B., Blomqvist, G., and Mitchell, J.H., *et al.:* Response to exercise after bed rest and after training. *Circulation, 38:* Suppl 12:1–55, 1968.

25. Siegel, W., Blomqvist, G., and Mitchell, J.H.: Effects of a quantitated physical training program on middle-aged sedentary men. *Circulation, 41:*19–29, 1970.

26. Grimby, G., and Saltin, B.: Physiological analysis of physically well trained middle-aged and old athletes. *Acta Med Scand, 179:*513–526, 1966.

27. Naughton, J., Shanbour, K., and Armstrong, R., et al.: Cardiovascular responses to exercise following myocardial infarction. *Arch Intern Med, 117:*541–545, 1966.

28. Varnauskas, E., Bergman, H., and Houk, P., et al.: Hemodynamic effects of physical training in coronary patients. *Lancet, 2:*8–12, 1966.

29. Frick, M.H., and Katila, M.: Hemodynamic consequences of physical training after myocardial infarction. *Circulation, 37:*192–202, 1968.

30. Clausen, J.P., and Trap-Jensen, J.: Effects of training on the distribution of cardiac output in patients with coronary artery disease. *Circulation, 42:*611–624, 1970.

31. Detry, J.M.R., Rousseau, M. and Vandenbroucke, G., *et al.:* Increased arteriovenous oxygen difference after physical training in coronary heart disease. *Circulation, 44:*109–118, 1971.

32. Siegel, W., Gilbert, C.A., and Nutter, D.O., *et al.:* Use of isometric handgrip for the indirect assessment of left ventricular function in patients with coronary atherosclerotic heart disease. *Am J Cardiol, 30:*48–54, 1972.

33. Lind, A.R.: Cardiovascular responses to static exercise (editorial). *Circulation 41:*173–176, 1970.

34. Wahren, J. and Bygdeman, S.: Onset of angina pectoris in relation to circulatory adaptation during arm and leg exercise. *Circulation, 44:* 432–441, 1971.

35. Sheffield, L.T., Roitman, D., and Reeves, T.J.: Hemodynamic consequences of physical training after myocardial infarction. *Circulation, 37:*192–202, 1968.

36. Frick, M.H., Elovainic, R.O., and Somer, T.: The mechanism of bradycardia evoked by physical training. *Cardiologia* (Basel), *51:*46–54, 1967.

*Chapter III*

37. Froelicher, V.F.: Animal studies of effect of chronic exercise on the heart and atherosclerosis: A review. *Am Heart J, 84:*496–506, 1972.

38. Bloor, C.M., Pasyk, S., and Leon, A.S.: Interaction of age and exercise on organ and cellular development. *Am. J Pathol, 58:*185–199, 1970.

39. Hakkila, J.: Studies of the myocardial capillary concentration in cardiac hypertrophy due to training. *Ann Med Exp Biol Fenn, 33:* Suppl 10:1, 1955.

40. Banister, E.W., Tomanek, R.J., and Cvorkov, N.: Ultrastructural modifications in rat heart: Responses to exercise and training. *Am. J Physiol, 220:*1935–1940, 1971.

41. Poupa, O., Rakusan, K., and Ostadal, B.: The effect of physical activity upon the heart of vertebrates. In Brunner, E., (Ed.) : Physical activity and aging. *Med Sports, 4:*202, 1970.

42. Leon, A.S., and Bloor, C.M.: Exercise effects on the heart at different ages (Abstr) . *Circulation, 41* and *42* (Suppl III) :50, 1970.

43. Tomanek, R.J.: Effects of age and exercise on the extent of the myocardial capillary bed. *Anat Rec, 167:*55–62, 1970.

44. Poupa, O., Rakusan, K., and Ostadal, B.: The effect of physical activity upon the heart of vertebrates. In Brunner, E., (Ed.) : Physical activity and aging. *Med Sports, 4:*202, 1970.

45. Eckstein, R.W.: Effect of exercise and coronary artery narrowing on coronary collateral circulation. *Circ Res, 5:*230–235, 1957.

46. Cobb, F.R., Ruby, R.L., and Fariss, B.L.: Effects of exercise on acute coronary occlusion in dogs with prior partial occlusion (Abstr.) . *Circulation, 37* and *38:*104, 1968.

47. Burt, J.J., and Jackson, R.: The effects of physical exercise on the coronary collateral circulation of dogs. *J Sports Med, 5:*203–206, 1965.

48. Kaplinsky, E., Hood, W.B., Jr., and McCarthy, B., *et al.:* Effects of physical training in dogs with coronary artery ligation. *Circulation, 37:*556–565, 1968.

49. Tepperman, J., and Pearlman, D.: Effects of exercise and anemia on coronary arteries of small animals as revealed by the corrosion-case technique: *Circ Res, 9:*576–584, 1961.

50. Stevenson, J.A.F., Feleki, V., and Rechnitzer, P., *et al.:* Effect of exercise on coronary tree size in the rat. *Circ Res, 5:*265, 1964.
51. Penpargkul, S., and Scheuer, J.: The effect of physical training upon the mechanical and metabolic performance of the rat heart. *J Clin Invest, 49:*1859–1868, 1970.
52. Holloszy, J.O.: Morphological and enzymatic adaptations to training: A review. In Larsen, O.A., and Malmborg, R.O., (Ed.) : *Coronary heart disease and physical fitness.* University Park Press, Baltimore, 1971, 147–151.
53. Arcos, J.C., Sohal, R.S., and Sun, S.C., *et al.:* Changes in ultra-constructure and respiratory control in mitochondria of rat heart hypertrophied by exercise. *Exp Molec Pathol, 8:*49–65, 1968.
54. Aldinger, E.E., and Sohol, R.S.: Effects of digitoxin on the ultrastructural myocardial changes in the rat subjected to chronic exercise. *Am J Cardiol, 26:*369–374, 1970.
55. Froelicher, V.F., and Oberman, A.: Analysis of epidemiologic studies of physical inactivity as risk factor for coronary artery disease. *Prog Cardiovasc Dis, 15:*41–65, 1972.
56. Morris, J.N., Heady, J.A., and Raffle, P.A., *et al.:* Coronary heart disease and physical activity of work. *Lancet, 2:*1053–1057, 1953.
57. Morris, J.N., Kagan, A., and Pattison, D.C., *et al.:* Incidence and prediction of ischemic heart disease in London busmen. *Lancet, 2:*553–559, 1966.
58. Taylor, H.L., Klepetar, E., and Keys, A., *et al.:* Death rate among physically active and sedentary employees of the railroad industry. *Am J Publ Health, 52:*1697, 1962.
59. Taylor, H.L., Blackburn, H., and Brozek, J., *et al.:* Occupational factors in the study of coronary heart disease and physical activity. *Can Med Assoc J, 96:*825, 1967.
60. Frank, C.W., Weinblatt, E., and Shapiro, S., *et al.:* Physical inactivity as a lethal factor in myocardial infarction among men. *Circulation, 34:*1022–1033, 1966.
61. Keys, A.: Physical activity and the epidemiology of coronary heart disease. In Brunner, D. (Ed.) : Physical activity and aging. *Medicine and Sport,* Vol. 4, Baltimore, University Park Press, 250, 1970.
62. McDonough, J.R., Hames, C.G., and Stubb, S.C., *et al.:* Coronary heart disease among Negroes and Whites in Evans County, Georgia. *J Chronic Dis 18:*443, 1965.
63. Hames, C.G.: Evans County cardiovascular and cerebrovascular epidemiology study: Introduction. *Arch Intern Med, 128:*883–886, 1971.
64. Pomeroy, W.C., and White, P.D.: Coronary heart disease in former football players. *JAMA, 167:*711–714, 1958.
65. Prout, C.: Life expectancy of college oarsmen. *JAMA, 220:*1709–1711, 1972.

66. Schnohr, P.: Longevity and causes of death in male athletic champions. *Lancet, 2:*1364–1366, 1971.

67. Polednak, A.P.: Longevity and cardiovascular mortality among former college athletes. *Circulation, 46:*649–654, 1972.

68. Kannel, W.B.: Habitual level of physical activity and risk of coronary heart disease: The Framingham study. *Can Med Assoc J, 96:*811–812, 1967.

69. Paffenbarger, R.S., Laughlin, M.E., and Gima, A.S., *et al.:* Work activity of longshoremen as related to death from coronary heart disease and stroke. *N Engl J Med, 282:*1109, 1970.

70. Blackburn, H., Taylor, H.L., and Keys, A.: Coronary heart disease in seven countries. XVI. The electrocardiogram in prediction of five-year coronary heart disease incidence among men aged 40–59. *Circulation, 41* (Suppl 1) :154, 1970.

71. Werko, L.: Can we prevent heart disease. *Ann Intern Med, 74:*278–288, 1971.

72. Morris, J.N., Adam, C., and Chave, S.P.W., *et al.:* Vigorous exercise in leisuretime and the incidence of coronary heart disease. *Lancet, 1:* 333–339, 1973.

73. Morris, J.N., Heady, J.A., and Raffle, P.A.B., *et al.:* Coronary heart disease and physical activity of work. *Lancet, 2:*1053–1057, 1953.

74. Gottheiner, V.: Long range strenuous sports training for cardiac reconditioning and rehabilitation. *Am J Cardiol, 22:*426–435, 1968.

75. Hellerstein, H.K.: The effects of physical activity: Patients and normal coronary-prone subjects. *Minn Med, 52:*1335–1341, 1969.

76. Rechnitzer, P.A., Pickard, H.A., and Paivio, A.U., *et al.:* Long-term follow-up study of survival and recurrence rates following myocardial infarction in exercising and control subjects. *Circulation, 45:*853–857, 1972.

77. Leaf, A.: Every day is a gift when you are over 100. *Natl Geographic, 143:*93–119, 1973.

78. Zukel, W.J., *et al.:* A short-term community study of the epidemiology of coronary heart disease. *Am J Public Health, 49:*1630, 1959.

79. Stamler, J., Lindberg, H.A., and Berkson, D.M., *et al.:* Prevalence and incidence of coronary heart disease in strata of the labor force of a Chicago industrial corporation. *J Chronic Dis, 11:*405–420, 1960.

Chapter IV

80. Dawber, T.R., and Kannel, W.B.: Susceptibility to coronary heart disease. *Mod Concepts Cardiovasc Dis, 30:*671–676, 1961.

81. Doyle, J.T.: Etiology of coronary disease: Risk factors influencing coronary disease. *Mod Concepts Cardiovasc Dis, 35:*81–86, 1966.

82. Stamler, J., Berkson, D.M., and Lindberg, H.A., *et al.:* Coronary risk factors: Their impact and their therapy in the prevention of coronary heart disease. *Med Clin N Am, 50:*229–254, 1966.

83. Ostrander, L.D., Jr.: Alternations of factors predisposing to coronary heart disease. *Ann Intern Med, 68:*1072–1077, 1968.

84. Rosenman, R.H., Friedman, M., and Straus, R., *et al.:* A predictive study of coronary disease. *JAMA, 189:*15 22, 1964.

85. Trulson, M.F., Clancy, R.E., and Jessop, W.J., *et al.:* Comparisons of siblings in Boston and Ireland. *J Am Diet Assoc, 45:*225–229, 1964.

86. Mann, G.V., Shaffer, R.D., and Rich, A.: Physical fitness and immunity to heart disease in Masai. *Lancet, 2:*1308–1310, 1965.

87. McDonough, J.R., Hames, C.G., and Stubb, S.C., *et al.:* Coronary heart disease among Negroes and Whites in Evans County, Georgia. *J Chronic Dis, 18:*443, 1965.

88. Shaper, A.G., and Jones, K.W.: Serum-cholesterol in camel-herding nomads. *Lancet, 2:*1305–1307, 1962.

89. Cantwell, J.D.: Coronary heart disease in young prisoners. Unpublished data.

90. Walker, W. J., and Gregoratos, G.: Myocardial infarction in young men. *Am J Cardiol, 19:*339–343, 1967.

91. Keys, A.: Coronary heart disease in seven countries. *Circulation, 41:* Suppl 1:1–198, 1970.

92. Fredrickson, D.S., Levy, R.I., and Lees, R.S.: Fat transport in lipoproteins—An integrated approach to mechanisms and disorders. *N Engl J Med, 276:*215–225, 1967.

93. Myasnikov, A.L.: Influence of some factors on development of experimental cholesterol atherosclerosis. *Circulation, 17:*99–113, 1958.

94. Kobernick, S.D., Niawayama, G., and Zuehlewski, A.C.: Effect of physical activity on cholesterol atherosclerosis in rabbits. *Proc Soc Exp Biol Med, 96:*623, 1957.

95. Montoye, H.J.: Summary of research on the relationship of exercise to heart disease. *J Sports Med, 2:*35–43, 1962.

96. Gollnick, P.D.: Cellular adaptation to exercise. In Shepard, R.J. (Ed.) : *Frontiers of Fitness,* Springfield, Thomas, 1971, p. 122.

97. Watt, E.W., Foss, M.L., and Block, W.D.: Effects of training and detraining on the distribution of cholesterol, triglyceride, and nitrogen in tissues of Albino Rats. *Circ Res, 31:*908–914, 1972.

98. Dalderup, L.M., Voogd, N. de, and Meyknecht, E.A., *et al.:* The effects of increasing the daily physical activity on the serum cholesterol levels. *Nutr Dieta,* (Basel) , *9:*112–123, 1967.

99. Hoffman, A.A., Nelson, W.R., and Goss, F.A.: Effects of an exercise program on plasma lipids of senior air force officers. *Am J Cardiol, 20:*516–524, 1967.

100. Clausen, J.P., Larse, N.O.A., and Trap-Jensen, J.: Physical training in the management of coronary artery disease. *Circulation, 40:*143–154, 1969.

101. Mann, G.V., Garrett, H.L., Farhi, A., Murray, H., and Billings, F.T.: Exercise to prevent coronary heart disease. An experimental study of

the effects of training on risk factors for coronary disease in men. *Am J Med, 46*:12–27, 1969.

102. Campbell, D.E.: Effect of controlled running on serum cholesterol of young adult males of varying morphological constitutions. *Res Q Am Assoc Health Phys Educ, 39*:47–53, 1968.

103. Berkson, D., *et al.*: Experience with a long-term supervised ergometric exercise program for middle-aged sedentary American men. *Circulation, 36*:Suppl 2:67, 1967.

104. Mann, G.V., *et al.*: Exercise and coronary risk factors: *Circulation, 36:* Suppl 2:181, 1967.

105. Golding, L.A.: Effects of exercise training upon total serum cholesterol levels. *Res Q Am Assoc Health Phys Educ, 33:*499, 1961.

106. Johnson, T.F., *et al.*: The influence of exercise on serum cholesterol, phospholipids, and electrophoretic serum protein patterns in college swimmers. *Fed Proc, 18:*77, 1959.

107. Karvonen, M.J., *et al.*: Serum cholesterol of male and female champion skiers. *Ann Med Int Fenn, 47:*75, 1958.

108. Chailley-Bert, Libignette, P., and Fabre-Chevalier: Contribution a L'Tude des variations du cholesterol sanguin au corns des achivities physique. *La Presse Medicale, 63:*415–416, 1955.

109. Rochelle, R.H.: Blood plasma cholesterol changes during a physical training program. *Am Assoc Health Phys Educ, 32:*838, 1961.

110. Phillips, L.: Physical fitness changes in adults attributable to equal periods of training, non-training, and re-training. Doctoral Dissertation, University of Illinois, 1960.

111. Daniel, B.J.: The effects of walking, jogging and running on the serum lipid concentration of the adult Caucasian male. Doctoral Dissertation, Univ. of Southern Mississippi, 1969.

112. Pollock, M.L., *et al.*: Effects of frequency of training on serum lipids, cardiovascular function, and body composition. In Franks, B. Don (Ed.) : *Exercise and Fitness. Chicago,* Athletic Institute, 1969, p. 161.

113. Konttinen, A.: Frysinen Akstiviteeti ja Seerumia Lipidit. *Sotiaslaatietillinen Aikakauslchti, 35:*169, 1960.

114. Pohndorf, R.H.: Improvements in physical fitness on two middle-aged adults. Doctoral Dissertation, University of Illinois, 1957.

115. Metivier, J.G.: The effects of five different physical exercise programs on the blood serum cholesterol of adult women. Doctoral Dissertation, University of Illinois, 1960.

116. Calvy, G.L., Cady, L.D., Mufson, M.A., Nierman, J., and Gertler, M.M.: Serum lipids and enzymes. Their levels after high-caloric, high-fat intake and vigorous exercise regimen in marine corps recruit personnel. *JAMA, 183:*1–4, 1963.

117. Holloszy, J.O., Skinner, J.S., and Toto, G.: Effects of a six-month program of endurance exercise on the serum lipids of middle-aged men. *Am J Cardiol, 14:*753–760, 1964.

118. Karvonen, M.W.: Effects of vigorous exercise on the heart. In Rosenbaum, F.F., and Belknap, E.L. (Eds.) : *Work and the Heart.* New York, Paul B. Hoebner, Inc., 1959, p. 190.

119. Skinner, J.S.: The effect of an endurance exercise program on the serum lipids of middle-aged men. PhD Dissertation, University of Illinois, 1963.

120. Olson, H.W.: The effect of supervised exercise program on the blood cholesterol of middle-aged men. *Physical Education, 15:*135, 1958.

121. Brumbach, W.B.: Changes in the serum cholesterol levels of male college students who participated in vigorous physical exercise program. Doctoral Dissertation, University of Oregon, 1959.

122. Zauner, C.W., and Swenson, E.W.: Physical training performance in relation to blood lipid levels and pulmonary function. *Am Correct Ther J, 21:*159, 1967.

123. Rochelle, R.: Blood plasma cholesterol changes during a physical training program. *Res Am Assoc Health Phys Educ, 32:*538, 1961.

124. Romanova, D., and Barbarin, P.: The influence of physical exercises on the content of serum protein, lipoprotein and total cholesterol in persons of middle and elderly age with symptoms of atherosclerosis. *Kardiologiia, 1:*36, 1961.

125. Mirkin, G.: Labile serum cholesterol values. *N Engl J Med, 279:*1001, 1968.

126. Oscai, L.B., Patterson, J.A., Bogard, D.L., *et al.:* Normalization of serum triglycerides and lipoprotein electrophoretic patterns by exercise. *Am J Cardiol, 30:*775–780, 1972.

127. Nikkila, E.A., and Konttinen, A.: Effect of physical activity on postprandial levels of fats in serum. *Lancet, 1:*1151–1154, 1962.

128. Cohen, H., and Goldberg, C.: Effect of physical exercise on alimentary lipaemia. *Br Med J, 5197:*509–511, 1960.

129. Varnauskas, E., Bergman, H., and Houk, P.: Haemodynamic effects of physical training in coronary patients. *Lancet, 2:*8–12, 1966.

130. Goode, R.C., Firstbrook, J.B., and Shephard, R.J.: Effects of exercise and cholesterol-free diet on human serum lipids. *Can J Physiol Pharmacol, 44:*575–580, 1966.

131. Taylor, H.L.: Occupational factors in the study of coronary heart disease and physical activity. *Can Med Assoc J, 96:*825–831, 1967.

132. Kang, B.S., Song, S.J., and Suh, C.S., *et al.:* Changes in body temperature and basal metabolic rate. *Amer J Appl Physical, 18:*483–488, 1963.

133. Miall, W.E., and Oldham, P.D.: Factors influencing arterial blood pressure in the general population. *Clin Sci, 17:*409–444, 1958.

134. Karvonen, M.J., Rantaharun, P.M., and Orma, S., *et al.:* Cardiovascular studies on lumberjacks. *J Occup Med, 3:*49–53, 1961.

135. Morris, J.N.: Epidemiology and cardiovascular disease of middle age: Part II. *Mod Concepts Cardiovasc Dis, 30:*633–638, 1960.

136. Keys, A., Aravanis, C., and Blackburn, H.W., *et al.:* Epidemiological studies related to coronary heart disease: Characteristics of men aged 40–59 in Seven Countries. *Acta Med Scand* Suppl, 460, 1966.

137. Chiang, B.N., Alexander, E.R., and Bruce, R.A., *et al.:* Physical characteristics and exercise performance of pedicab and upper socioeconomic classes of middle-aged Chinese men. *Am Heart J, 76:*760–768, 1968.

138. Doan, A.E., Peterson, D.R., and Blackman, J.R., *et al.:* Myocardial ischemia after maximal exercise in healthy men. *Am J Cardiol, 17:* 9–19, 1966.

139. Berkson, D.M., Stamler, J., and Lindberg, H.A., *et al.:* Socioeconomic correlates of atherosclerotic and hypertensive heart disease. *Ann NY Acad Sci, 84:*835–850, 1960.

140. Raab, W., and Krzywanek, H. J.: Cardiovascular sympathetic tone and stress response related to personality patterns and exercise habits. *Am J Cardiol, 16:*42–53, 1965.

141. Rose, G.: Physical activity and coronary heart disease. *Proc R Soc Med, 62:*1183–1188, 1969.

142. Montoye, H.J., Metzner, H.L., and Keller, J.B., *et al.:* Habitual physical activity and blood pressure. *Med Sci Sports, 4:*175–181, Winter, 1972.

143. Harris, W.E., Bowerman, W., and McFadden, R.B., *et al.:* Jogging, An adult exercise program. *JAMA, 201:*759–761, 1967.

144. Boyer, J.L., and Kasch, F.W.: Exercise therapy in hypertensive men. *JAMA, 211:*1668–1671, 1970.

145. Mellerowicz, H.: Vergleichende Untersuchungen uber das Oknomieprinvip in Arbeit und Leistung des trainierten Kreislaufs und seine Bedeutung fur die preventive and rehabilitive Medizi. *Arch Kreislaufforsch, 24:*70, 1956.

146. Naughton, J., Shanbour, K., Armstrong, R., McCoy, J., and Lategola, M.T.: Cardiovascular responses to exercise following myocardial infarction. *Arch Int Med* (Chicago), *117:*541–545, 1966.

147. Pyorala, K., Karava, R., Punsar, S., *et al.:* A controlled study of the effects of 18 months physical training in sedentary middle-aged men with high indexes of risk relative to coronary heart disease. In *Larsen, O. Andree, and Malmborg, R.D., (Eds.): Coronary Heart Disease and Physical Fitness.* Munksgaard, 1971, p. 261.

148. Kentala, E.: Physical fitness and feasibility of physical rehabilitation after myocardial infarctions in men of working age. *Ann Clin Res 4,* Suppl 9:1–84, 1972.

149. Levine, S.A., Gordon, B., and Derick, C.L.: Some changes in the chemical constituents of the blood following a marathon race with special reference to the development of hypoglycemia. *JAMA, 82:*1778–1779, 1924.

150. Blotner, H.: Effect of prolonged physical inactivity on tolerance of sugar. *Arch Intern Med, 75:*39–44, 1945.

151. Davidson, P.C., Shane, S.R., and Albrink, M.J.: Decreased glucose tolerance following a physical conditioning program. *Circulation, 34,* Suppl 3:7, 1966.

152. Mayer, J.: Some aspects of the problem of regulation of food intake and obesity. *N Engl J Med, 274:*662–673, 1966.

153. Nelson, R.A., Anderson, L.F., and Gastineau, C.F., *et al.:* Physiology and natural history of obesity. *JAMA, 223:*627–630, 1973.

154. Frick, M.H.: The effect of physical training in manifest ischemic heart disease. *Circulation, 40:*433–435, 1969.

155. Skinner, J.S., Holloszy, J.O., and Cureton, T.K.: Effects of a program of endurance exercises on physical work. *Am J Cardiol, 14:*747–752, 1964.

156. Rechnitzer, P.A., Yuhasz, M.S., and Pickard, H.A., *et al.:* Effects of a 24-week exercise program on normal adults and patients with previous myocardial infarction. *Br Med J, 1:*734–735, 1967.

157. Morris, J.N., Heady, J.A., and Raffle, P.A.B., *et al.:* Coronary heart disease and physical activity of work. *Lancet, 2:*1053–1057, 1953.

158. Boileau, R.A., Buskirk, E.R., and Horstman, D.H., *et al.:* Body composition changes in obese and lean men during physical conditioning. *Med Sci Sports, 3:*183–189, 1971.

159. McPherson, B.D., Paivo, A., Yuhasz, M.S., *et al.:* Psychological effects of an exercise program for post-infarction and normal adult men. *J Sports Med, 7:*3, 1967.

160. Ismail, A.H., and Trachtman, L.E.: Jogging the imagination. *Psychology Today, 7:*79–82, 1973.

161. Hellerstein, H.K.: Exercise therapy in coronary disease. *Bull NY Acad Med, 44:*1028–1047, 1968.

162. Naughton, J., Bruhn, J.G., and Lategola, M.T.: Effects of physical training on physiological and behavioral characteristics of cardiac patients. *Arch Phys Med, 49:*131, 1968.

163. Hellerstein, H.K., and Friedman, E.H.: Sexual activity and the post coronary patient. *Medical Aspects of Human Sexual, 3:*70, 1969.

164. Hellerstein, H.K., and Friedman, E.H.: Sexual activity and the post-coronary patient. *Arch. Intern Med, 125:*987–999, 1970.

165. Baekeland, F.: Exercise deprivation. *Arch Gen Psychiat, 22:*365–369, 1970.

166. Chiang, B.N., Perlman, L.V., Ostrander, L.D., and Epstein, F.H.: Relationship of premature systoles to coronary heart disease and sudden death in the Tecumseh epidemiologic studies. *Ann Intern Med, 70:*1159–1166, 1969.

167. Rotman, M., Colvard, M.D., and Ruskin, J., *et al.:* Nonspecific T-wave changes. *Arch Intern Med, 130:*895–897, 1972.

168. Kannel, W.B., Gordon, T., and Castelli, W.P., *et al.:* Electrocardiographic left ventricular hypertrophy and risk of coronary heart disease. *Ann Intern Med, 72:*813–822, 1970.

169. Smith, W.G., Cullen, K.G., and Thorburn, I.O.: Electrocardiograms of marathon runners in 1962 Commonwealth games. *Br Heart J, 26:* 469–476, 1964.

170. Spann, J.F., Jr., Mason, D.T., and Zelis, R.F.: Recent advances in the understanding of congestive heart failure. *Mod Concepts Cardiovasc Dis, 39:*73–78, 1970.

171. Hellerstein, H.K., Hirsch, E.Z., and Cumber, W., et al.: Reconditioning of the coronary patient: A preliminary report. In Likoff, W., and Moyer, J.G. (Eds.): *Coronary Heart Disease.* New York, Grune & Stratton, 1963, p. 448–454.

172. Burt, J.J., et al.: The effects of exercise on the coagulation-fibrinolysis equilibrium. U.S. Naval Medical Field Research Laboratory, Camp LeJune, N.C., 1962.

173. MacDonald, G.A., and Fullerton, H.W.: Effects of physical activity on increased coagulation of blood after ingesting high-fat meal. *Lancet,* 2:1006, 1971.

174. Warnock, N.H., et al.: Effects of exercise on blood coagulation time and atherosclerosis of cholesterol-fed cockerels. *Circ Res, 5:*478, 1957.

175. Iatridis, S.G., and Ferguson, J.H.: Effects of physical exercise on blood clotting and fibrinolysis. *J Appl Physiol, 18:*337–344, 1963.

176. Egeberg, O.: The effect of exercise on the blood clotting system. *Scand J Clin Lab Invest, 15:*8–13, 1963.

177. McDonald, G.A., and Fullterton, H.W.: Comparison of animal and vegetable fats in increasing blood coagulability. *Lancet,* 2:598–599, 1958.

178. Guest, M.M., and Celander, D.R.: Fibrinolytic activity in exercise. *Physiologist, 3:*69, 1960.

179. Astrup, T., and Brakman, P.: Responders and non-responders in exercise-induced blood fibrinolysis. In Larsen, O.A., and Malmborg, R. D. (Ed.): *Coronary Heart Disease and Physical Fitness.* Baltimore, University Park Press, 1971, p. 130.

180. Buzina, R., and Keys, A.: Blood coagulation after a fat meal. *Circulation, 14:*854–858, 1956.

181. McDonald, L., and Edgill, M.: Coagulability of the blood in ischemic heart disease. *Lancet,* 2:457–460, 1957.

182. Montoye, H. J., Howard, G.E., and Wood, J.H.: Observations of some hemochemical and anthropometric measurements in athletes. *J Sports Med, 7:*35–44, 1967.

183. Bosco, J.S., Greenleaf, J.E. and Kaye, R.L.: Reduction of serum uric acid in young men during physical training. *Am J Cardiol, 25:*46–52, 1970.

184. Dawber, T.R.: Identification of excess cardiovascular risk. A practical approach. *Minn Med, 52:*1217–1221, 1969.

185. Rechnitzer, P.A., Yuhasz, M.S., and Pickard, H.A., et al.: The effects of

a graduated exercise program on patients with previous myocardial infarction. *Can Med Assoc J, 92:*858–860, 1965.

186. Lefcoe, N.M., and Paterson, N.A.M.: Adjunct therapy in chronic obstructive pulmonary disease. *Am J Med, 54:*343–349, 1973.

*Chapter V*

187. Feil, H., and Siegel, M.L.: Electrocardiographic changes during attacks of angina. *Am J Med Sci, 175:*256, 1928.

188. Master, A.M., and Oppenheimer, E.T.: A simple tolerance test for circulatory efficiency with standard tables for normal individuals. *Am J Med Sci, 177:*223–242, 1929.

189. Scherf, D., and Goldhammer, S.: Zur frubdiagnose der angina pectoris mit helfe des eletrokarkograms. *Z Klin Med, 124:*111, 1933.

190. Astrand, P.O., and Rodahl, K.: *Textbook of Work Physiology.* New York, McGraw-Hill, 1970.

191. Master, A.M.: Exercise testing for evaluation of cardiac performance. *Am J Cardiol, 30:*718–721, 1972.

192. Cohen, P.F., Vokonas, P.S., and Most, A.S., *et al.:* Diagnostic accuracy of two-step post-exercise ECG. Result in 305 subjects studied by coronary arteriography. *JAMA, 220:*501–506, 1972.

193. Fletcher, G.F.: Submaximal treadmill exercise evaluation in patients with symptoms of cardiovascular disease. *Chest, 63:*153–158, 1973.

194. Doan, A.E., Peterson, D.R., and Blackmon, J.R., *et al:* Myocardial ischemia after maximal exercise in healthy men. A method for detecting potential coronary heart disease? *Am Heart J, 69:*11–21, 1965.

195. Most, A.S., Hornstein, T.R., and Hofer, V., *et al.:* Exercise S-T changes in healthy men. *Arch Intern Med, 121:*225–229, 1968.

196. Spangler, R.D., Horman, M.J., and Miller, S.W., *et al.:* A submaximal exercise electrocardiographic test as a method of detecting occult ischemic heart disease. *Am Heart J, 80:*752–758, 1970.

197. Ellestad, M.H., Allen, W., and Wan, M.C., *et al.:* Maximal treadmill stress testing for cardiovascular evaluation. *Circulation, 39:*517–522, 1969.

198. Fox, S.M., III, Naughton, J.P., and Haskell, W.L.: Physical activity and the prevention of coronary heart disease. *Ann Clin Res, 3:*404–432, 1971.

199. Astrand, P.O., and Rodahl, K.: *Textbook of Work Physiology.* New York, McGraw-Hill Co., 1970, p. 362–363.

200. Shepard, R.V., Aleen, C., and Benade, A.V.S., *et al.:* The maximal oxygen intake. An international reference standard of cardiorespiratory fitness. *Bull WHO, 38:*757, 1968.

201. Bruce, R.A., Kusumi, F., and Hosmer, D.: Maximal oxygen intake and nomographic assessment of functional aerobic impairment in cardiovascular disease. *Am Heart J, 85:*546–562, 1973.

202. Mason, R.E., and Likar, I.: A new system of multiple-lead exercise electrocardiography. *Am Heart J, 71*:196–205, 1966.

203. Hellerstein, H.K., Hornstein, T.R., and Goldbarg, A.W., *et al.:* The influence of active conditioning upon coronary atherosclerosis. A progress report. In Brest, A.N., and Moyer, J.H., (Ed.) : *Atherosclerotic Vascular Disease.* New York, Appleton-Century-Crofts, 1967, p. 115.

204. Redwood, D.R., and Epstein, S.E.: Uses and limitations of stress testing in the evaluation of ischemic heart disease. *Circulation, 46*:1115–1131, 1972.

205. Sheffield, L.T., Roitman, D., and Reeves, T.J.: Submaximal exercise testing. *J SC Med Assoc, 65*, Suppl 1:18–25, 1969.

206. Summation of guidelines on exercise. *J SC Assoc, 65*:92, 1969.

207. Cumming, G.R.: Yield of ischemic exercise electrocardiograms in relation to exercise intensity in a normal population. *Br Heart J, 34*: 919–923, 1972.

208. Wood, P.C., and Wolfeth, C.C.: Angina pectoris; clinical and electrocardiographic phenomena of attack and their comparison with effects of experimental temporary coronary occlusion. *Arch Intern Med, 47*:339, 1931.

209. Mattingly, T.W.: The post-exercise electrocardiogram. *Am J Cardiol, 9*:395–409, 1962.

210. Brody, A.J.: Master two-step exercise test in clinically unselected patients. *JAMA, 171*:1195–1198, 1959.

211. Doyle, J.T., and Kinch, S.H.: The prognosis of an abnormal electrocardiographic stress test. *Circulation, 41*:545–553, 1970.

212. Beard, E.F., Garcia, E., and Burke, G.E., *et al.:* Postexercise electrocardiogram in screening for latent ischemic heart disease. *Dis Chest, 56:* 405–408, 1969.

213. Kattus, A.A., Jorgensen, C.R., and Worden, R.E., *et al.:* S-T-segment depression with near-maximal exercise in detection of preclinical coronary heart disease. *Circulation, 44*:585–595, 1971.

214. Blackburn, H.W., Taylor, H.L., and Keys, A.: Prognostic significance of the postexercise electrocardiogram: Risk factors held constant. *Am J Cardiol, 25*:85, 1970.

215. Robb, G.P., and Marks, H.H.: Postexercise electrocardiogram in arteriosclerotic heart disease: Its value in diagnosis and prognosis. *JAMA, 171*:1195, 1959.

216. Bellet, S., Roman, L.R., and Nichols, G.J., *et al.:* Detection of the coronary-prone subjects in a normal population by radioelectrocardiographic exercise test: Follow-up studies. *Am J Cardiol, 19*:783–787, 1967.

217. Aronow, W.S.: Thirty-month follow-up of maximal treadmill stress test and double Master's tests in normal subjects. *Circulation, 47*:287–290, 1973.

218. Mason, R.E., Likar, I., and Biern, R.O., *et al.:* Multiple-lead exercise electrocardiography: Experience in 107 normal subjects and 67 patients with angina pectoris, and comparison with coronary cineararteriography in 84 patients. *Circulation, 36:*517–525, 1967.

219. McConahay, D.R., McCallister, B.D., and Smith, R.E.: Postexercise electrocardiography: Correlations with coronary arteriography and left ventricular hemodynamics. *Am J Cardiol, 28:*1, 1971.

220. Martin, C.M., and McConahay, D.R.: Maximal treadmill exercise electrocardiography: Correlations with coronary arteriography and cardiac hemodynamics. *Circulation, 46:*956–962, 1972.

221. Lewis, W.J., and Wilson, W.J.: Correlation of coronary arteriograms with Master's test and treadmill test. *Rocky Mt Med J, 68:*30–34, 1972.

222. McHenry, P.L., Phillips, J.F., and Knoebel, S.B.: Correlation of the computer-quantitated treadmill exercise electrocardiogram with arteriographic location of coronary artery disease. *Am J Cardiol, 30:* 747–752, 1972.

223. Most, A.S., Kemp, H.G., and Gorlin, R.: Postexercise electrocardiography in patients with arteriographically documented coronary artery disease. *Ann Int Med, 71:*1043–1049, 1969.

224. Roitman, D., Jones, W.B., and Sheffield, L.T.: Comparison of submaximal exercise ECG test with coronary cineangiocardiogram. *Ann Intern Med, 72:*641–647, 1970.

225. Fortuin, N.J., and Friesinger, G.C.: Exercise-induced S-T segment elevation. *Amer J Med, 49:*459–464, 1970.

226. Weissler, A.M., Harris, W.S., and Schoenfeld, C.D.: Systolic time intervals in heart failure in man. *Circulation, 37:*149–159, 1968.

227. Garrard, C.L., Jr., Weissler, A.M., and Dodge, H.T.: Relationship of alterations in systolic time intervals to ejection fraction in patients with cardiac disease. *Circulation, 42:*455, 1970.

228. Pouget, J.M., Harris, W.S., and Myron, B.R., *et al.:* Abnormal responses of the systolic time intervals to exercise in patients with angina pectoris. *Circulation, 43:*289–298, 1971.

229. Whitsett, T.L., and Naughton, J.: The effect of exercise on systolic time intervals in sedentary and active individuals and rehabilitated patients with heart disease. *Am J Cardiol, 27:*352–358, 1971.

230. McConahay, D.R., Martin, C.M., and Cheitlin, M.D.: Resting and exercise systolic time intervals. Correlations with ventricular performance in patients with coronary artery disease. *Circulation, 45:*592–601, 1972.

231. Gilbert, C.G., and Cantwell, J.D.: The response of systolic time intervals following exercise in patients with coronary atherosclerotic heart disease (abstr). *Med Sci Sports, 4:*56–57, 1972.

232. Benchimol, A., and Dimond, E.G.: The apexcardiogram in normal

older subjects and in patients with arteriosclerotic heart disease. Effect of exercise on the "a" wave. *Am Heart J, 65*:789–801, 1963.

233. Aronow, W.S., Uyeyama, R.R., and Cassidy, J., *et al.:* Resting and post-exercise phonocardiograms and electrocardiograms in patients with angina pectoris and in normal subjects. *Circulation, 43*:273–278, 1971.

234. Feigenbaum, H.: Clinical applications of echocardiography *Prog Cardiovasc Dis, 14*:531–558, 1972.

235. Zaret, B.L., Strauss, H.W., and Martin, N.D., *et al.:* Noninvasive regional myocardial perfusion with radioactive potassium. *N Eng J Med, 288*:809–812, 1973.

236. Goldschlager, N., Cake, D. and Cohn, K.: Exercise-induced ventricular arrhythmias in patients with coronary heart disease. Their relation to angiographic findings. *Am J Cardiol, 31*:434–440, 1973.

237. Gooch, A.S.: Exercise testing for detecting changes in cardiac rhythm and conduction. *Am J Cardiol, 30*:741–746, 1972.

238. Vedin, J.A., Wilhelmsson, C.E., and Wilhelmsen, L., *et al.:* Relation of resting and exercise-induced ectopic beats to other ischemic manifestations and to coronary risk factors. *Am J Cardiol, 30*:25–31, 1972.

239. Singer, E., Gooch, A.S., and Morse, D.: Exercise-induced arrhythmias in patients with pacemakers. *JAMA, 224*:1515–1518, 1973.

240. Garrison, G.E., Floyd, W.L., and Orgain, E.S.: Exercise in the physical examination of peripheral arterial disease. *Ann Int Med, 66*:587–593, 1967.

241. Siegel, W., Attar, O.A., and Proudfit, W.L., *et al.:* Acute hemodynamic and clinical effects of direct coronary revascularization (Abstr.). *Am J Cardiol, 31*:158, 1973.

242. Kavanagh, T.: Application of exercise testing to elderly amputee. *Can Med Assoc J, 108*:314–318, 1973.

243. Mac Alpin, R.N., Kattus, A.A., and Alvaro, A.B.: Angina pectoris at rest with preservation of exercise capacity. Prinzmetal's variant angina. *Circulation, 47*:956, 1973.

244. Murray, J.A.: Exercise testing in the diagnosis of coronary artery disease. Luncheon Panel #9. American College of Cardiology. Washington, DC. Feb. 4, 1971.

245. Harris, C.N., Aronow, W.S., and Parker, D.P., *et al.:* Treadmill stress test in left ventricular hypertrophy. *Chest, 63*:353–357, 1973.

246. Riley, C.P., Oberman, A., and Sheffield, L.T.: Electrocardiographic effects of glucose ingestion. *Arch Intern Med, 130*:703–707, 1972.

247. Kaplan, M.A., Harris, C.N., and Aronow, W.S., *et al.:* Inability of the submaximal treadmill stress test to predict the location of coronary disease. *Circulation, 47*:250–255, 1973.

*Chapter VI*

248. Committee on Exercise and Physical Fitness: Evaluation for exercise

participation. The apparently healthy individual. *JAMA, 219:*900–901, 1972.

249. Fox, S.M., and Skinner, J.S.: Physical activity and cardiovascular health. *Am J Cardiol, 14:*731 746, 1964.

250. Cooper, K.H.: Guidelines in the management of the exercising patient. *JAMA, 211:*1663–1667, 1970.


*Chapter VII*

251. White, P.D.: Tardy growth of preventive cardiology. *Am J Cardiol, 29:* 886–888, 1972.

252. Page, I.H.: Atherosclerosis. A personal overview. *Circulation, 38:*1164–1172, 1968.

253. Cohn, P.F., Gorlin, R., and Vokonas, P.S., *et al.:* A quantitative clinical index for the diagnosis of symptomatic coronary-artery disease. *N Engl J Med, 286:*901–907, 1972.

254. Keys, A., Aravanis, C., and Blackburn, H., *et al.:* Probability of middle-aged men developing coronary heart disease in five years. *Circulation, 45:*815–828, 1972.


*Chapter VIII*

255. Levine, S.A., and Brown, D.L.: Coronary thrombosis: Its various clinical features. *Medicine* (Baltimore), *8:*245, 1929.

256. Coe, W.S.: Cardiac work and the chair treatment of acute coronary thrombosis. *Ann Int Med, 40:*42–48, 1954.

257. Mather, H.G., Pearson, N.G., and Read, K.L.Q., *et al.:* Acute myocardial infarction: Home and hospital treatment. *Br Med J, 3:*334–338, 1971.

258. Wenger, N.K., Hellerstein, H.K., and Blackburn, H., *et al.:* Uncomplicated myocardial infarction. Current physician practice in patient management. *JAMA, 224:*511–514, 1973.

259. Rose, G.: Early mobilization and discharge after myocardial infarction. *Mod Concepts Cardiovasc Dis, 41:*59–63, 1972.

260. Levine, S.A., and Lown, B.: Armchair treatment of acute coronary thrombosis. *JAMA, 148:*1365–1369, 1952.

261. Fareeduddin, K., and Abelmann, W.H.: Impaired orthostatic tolerance after bed rest in patients with myocardial infarction. *N Engl J Med, 280:*345–350, 1969.

262. Adgey, A.A.J.: Prognosis after early discharge from hospital of patients with acute myocardial infarction. *Br Heart J, 31:*750–752, 1969.

263. Takkunen, J., Huhti, E., and Oilinki, O., *et al.:* Early ambulation in myocardial infarction. *Acta Med Scand, 188:*103–106, 1970.

264. Tucker, H.H., Carson, P.H.M., and Bass, N.M., *et al.:* Results of early mobilization and discharge after myocardial infarction. *Br Med J, 1:*10–13, 1973.

265. Harpus, J.E., Conner, W.T., and Hamilton, M., *et al.:* Controlled trial

of early mobilization and discharge from hospital in uncomplicated myocardial infarction. *Lancet, 2*:1331–1334, 1971.

266. Hutter, A.M., Sidel, V.W., and Shine, K.I., *et al.:* Early hospital discharge after myocardial infarction. *N Engl J Med, 288*:1141–1144, 1973.

267. Wenger, N.K.: Physical activity, exercise testing, and exercise training programs for patients with myocardial infarction: The state of our knowledge (Editorial). *Acta Cardiol, 28*:13–17, 1973.

268. Browse, N.L.: Effect of bed rest on resting calf blood flow of healthy adult males. *Br Med J, 1*:1721–1723.

269. Makin, G.S., Mayes, F.B., and Holroyd, A.M.: Studies on the effect of "Tubigrip" on flow in the deep veins of the calf. *Br J Surg, 56*:369–372, 1929.

270. Rosengarten, D.S., Laird, J., and Jeyasingh, K., *et al.:* The failure of compression stockings (Tubigrip) to prevent deep venous thrombosis after operation. *Br J Surg, 57*:296–299, 1970.

271. Kakkar, V.V., Corrigan, T., and Spindler, J., *et al.:* Efficacy of low doses of heparin in prevention of deep vein thrombosis after major surgery: double-blind, randomized trial. *Lancet, 2*:101–106, 1972.

272. Handley, A.J.: Low-dose heparin after myocardial infarction. *Lancet, 2*:623–624, 1972.

273. Wray, R., Maurer, B., and Shillingford, J.: Prophylactic anticoagulant therapy in the prevention of calf-vein thrombosis after myocardial infarction. *N Engl J Med, 288*:815–817, 1973.

*Chapter IX*

274. Kennedy, C.C., Spiekerman, R.E., and Lindsey, M.I., *et al.:* Evaluation of a one-year graduated exercise program for men with angina pectoris by physiologic studies and coronary arteriography (Abstr.). *Am J Cardiol, 31*:141, 1973.

275. Ferguson, R.J., Choquette, G., and Chaniotis, L., *et al.:* Coronary arteriography and treadmill exercise capacity before and after 13 months physical training (Abstr.). *Med Sci Sports, 5*:67–68, 1973.

276. Kattus, A.A., Jr., Hanafee, W.N., and Longmire, W.P., Jr., *et al.:* Diagnosis, medical and surgical management of coronary insufficiency. *Ann Int Med, 69*:114–136, 1968.

277. Boyer, J.L.: Adult fitness starter program for individuals considered to be at high risk for coronary heart disease. *J SC Med Assoc, 65*, Suppl 1: 99, 1969.

278. Cooper, K.H.: *The New Aerobics.* New York, Evans and Co., 1970, p. 28.

279. Gallagher, J.R., Allman, F.L., Jr., and Guild, W.R., *et al.:* Is your patient fit? A simple supplementary test for evaluating a patient's fitness. *JAMA, 201*:117–118, 1967.

280. Sharrock, N., Garrett, H.L., and Mann, G.V.: Practical exercise test for

physical fitness and cardiac performance. *Am J Cardiol, 30:*727–732, 1972.

281. Stamler, J., Kjelsberg, M., and Hall, Y.: Epidemiologic studies on cardio-vascular-rcnal disease. *J Chronic Dis, 12:*440–455, 1960.

282. Fox, S.M., III, and Haskell, W.L.: Physical activity and the prevention of coronary heart disease. *Bull NY Acad Med, 44:*950–965, 1968.

283. Cantwell, J.D., and Fletcher, G.F.: Cardiac complications while jogging. *JAMA, 210:*130–131, 1969.

284. Parmley, L.F.: Proceedings of the National Conference on exercise in the prevention, in the evaluation, in the treatment of heart disease. *J SC Med Assoc, 65:*i, 1969.

285. Cohen, H.L.: Jogger's petechiae. *N Engl J Med, 279:*109, 1968.

286. Siegel, I.M.: Jogger's heel. *JAMA, 206:*2899, 1968.

287. Hunder, G.G.: Harmful effect of jogging. *Ann Intern Med, 71:*664–665, 1969.

288. Boyer, J.L.: Physical activity program following myocardial infarction. *Hosp Med, 8:*95–112, 1972.

289. Morgan, C.M.: Supervised training after myocardial infarction (Abstr.). *Br Heart J 34:*203, 1972.

290. Bowerman, W.J., Harris, W.E.: *Jogging.* New York, Grosset and Dunlap, Inc., 1967.

291. Stanley, E., and Kezdi, P.: Training variation in middle-aged males. *Circulation, 38, Suppl 6:*289, 1968.

292. Dawson, J.E., and Fletcher, G.F.: Treadmill exercise evaluation before and after an organized physical training program in a group of normal male executives. *Circulation,* Supplement to Vols XLIII and XLIV: 1175, 1971.

293. Fraser, R.S., and Chapman, C.B.: Studies on the effect of exercise on cardiovascular function; The blood pressure and pulse rate. *Circulation, 9:*193–198, 1954.

294. Logan, G.A., and Bruce, R.A.: A typical pressor responses to upright posture and exercise in patients with mitral or aortic stenosis. *Am J Med Sci, 236:*168–174, 1958.

295. Hiss, R.G., and Lamb, L.E.: Electrocardiographic findings in 122,043 individuals. *Circulation, 25:*947–961, 1962.

296. Lamb, L.E., and Hiss, R.G.: Influence of exercise on premature contractions. *Am J Cardiol, 10:*209–216, 1962.

297. Giese, W.K.: Exercise programs: Types, directions and dangers. *J SC Med Assoc, 65, Suppl I:*34–37, 1969.

298. Taylor, H.L., and Parlin, R.W.: The physical activity of railroad clerks and switchmen: estimation of on-the-job caloric expenditure by time and task measurements and classification of recreational activity by questionnaire. Presented at Three Days of Cardiology, June 25, 1966, at the University of Washington, Seattle.

299. Fox, S.M., III, and Haskell, W.L.: Physical activity and health maintenance. *J Rehab, 32*:89–92, 1966.

300. Hanson, S., Tabakin, B.S., and Levy, A.M., *et al.*: Long term physical training and cardiovascular dynamics in middle-aged men. *Circulation, 38*:783–799, 1968.

*Chapter XIII*

301. Wilhelmsen, L., Tibblin, G., and Werko, L.: A primary preventive study in Gothenburg, Sweden. *Prev Med, 1*:153–160, 1972.

302. Gustufson, A., Elmfeldt, D., and Wilhelmsen, L., *et al.*: Serum lipids and lipo-proteins in men after myocardial infarction compared with representative population sample. *Circulation, 46*:709–716, 1972.

303. Personal interview, April, 1973.

304. Stocksmeier, V.U., and Halhuber, M.J.: Die Hohenrieder langschnittstudie an herzinfarlg—patienten Munch. med Wschr, 114, p. 1349, 1972.

305. Paul, O.: The international cooperative study on epidemiology. *Circulation, 41*:895–897, 1970.

# AUTHOR INDEX

# SUBJECT INDEX